Pacemaker Interpretation for Nurses

*Everything you wanted to know about PACEMAKERS...
But didn't have time to look up!*

Carol J. V. O. Wallace, R.N.

Library of Congress catalog card number: 95-069076
ISBN 0-9627246-6-1

Printed in the United States of America

Design and Production: *Adam E. Blyn*

Published by:
Power Publications
56 McArthur Avenue
Staten Island, NY 10312
1-800-331-6534

Dedication

To Jeremy and Jonathan

Acknowledgements

I'd like to acknowledge my appreciation of the support, under-standing, and patience of Matthew T. Kuber, MD FACC who over the years has endured my many questions about pacemakers and also pro-vided me with much of the literature needed to complete this book.

Also, I appreciate the assistance of Richard Wallace in the prepa-ration of this book.

I'd like to thank Medtronic, Incorporated for their literature and for the assistance of their technical service department. Also, the ma-jority of rhythm strips presented in this book are actual rhythm strips from patient's with Medtronic pacemakers. The support of Medtronic, Incorporated is greatly appreciated.

Lastly, I appreciate the assistance of Intermedics Incorporated. Especially, their assistance in providing me with pacemaker rhythm strips. The examples of VVT pacing, AAI pacing, atrial pacing fol-lowed by intrinsic ventricular depolarization of a DDD pacemaker, loss of atrial capture, and crosstalk inhibiting ventricular pacing were pro-vided to me by Intermedics Incorporated.

Power Publications would like to thank Linda Jordan RN, CCRN for reviewing this book.

Table of Contents

Chapter 1

Introduction to Pacemakers

Purpose of Text

The purpose of this text is to present nurses with the basic information necessary to interpret pacemaker function from EKGs, rhythm strips, and pacemaker programming information.

Commonly seen pacemakers will be the focus of this text. Pacemakers with antitachycardia, defibrillation potential, or other rarely seen programmable features will not be discussed.

History of Pacemaker Implantation

The implantation of permanent pacemakers began in 1958. They were implanted surgically to treat symptomatic bradycardias and recurrent Stokes Adams attacks. Early pacemakers were single lead, single chamber devices that had no sensing ability. They simply paced the heart at a set rate. Since 1958 pacemaker technology has advanced rapidly. To state that today's pacemakers are complex is a gross understatement. Physicians today have a broad selection of pacemakers with many programmable features to choose from when deciding which pacemaker is best for their patients. Because of the diversity of pacemakers and current Medicare regulations, the decision to implant a permanent pacemaker can be difficult.

Today, patients with sick sinus syndrome, usually with symptomatic tachy-brady episodes, are the most frequent pacemaker recipients.

1

Other rhythm disturbances that benefit from pacemaker implantation are acquired symptomatic complete heart block, congenital complete heart block with symptomatic bradycardia, symptomatic Mobitz II AV block, sinus node dysfunction with or without tachyarrhythmias or AV block, and bradycardias associated with significant symptoms, such as dizziness, syncope, and hypotension. Also, patients with carotid sinus hypersensitivity benefit from pacemaker implantation.

The above dysrhythmias have one thing in common, they cause symptoms that will be alleviated by the increased stable heart rate provided by a pacemaker. Therefore, they are considered reasonable and necessary by Medicare and are eligible for Medicare and other insurers' coverage provided the condition is documented to be chronic or recurrent and not due to temporary conditions such as an acute myocardial infarction, drug side effect or toxicity, or electrolyte imbalance.

Due to the advancements in pacemaker technology, the number of patients with conditions that are treated with pacemakers are increasing, and nurses will be called upon to interpret pacemaker rhythms more frequently. This is a difficult task, considering that aside from cardiologists most medical professionals receive little formal education about pacemakers.

Pacemaker Implantation

Today pacing systems are generally implanted transvenously via the subclavian or jugular vein using local anesthetic. The physician advances the lead or leads to the heart via the superior vena cava. Generally, the lead is advanced to the apex of the right ventricle. If a dual chamber pacing system, also known as universal, AV sequential, or AV synchronous, is being utilized the physician advances a second, atrial lead, into the right atrium. The tip of the lead may be implanted in the atrial septum, atrial wall, atrial appendage, or rarely the coronary sinus. Leads are secured to the heart either actively with screw-in lead tips, a grasping jaw mechanism, or a helical coil to name a few methods, or passively by the proliferation of connective tissue around the lead with time. Active fixation is preferable because it provides immediate stability for the leads. Following the insertion of the lead or leads the physician obtains electrophysiologic (EP) information from the myocardium that is utilized to program the pacemaker.

For single lead pacing systems the physician determines the heart's threshold of stimulation. That is, the minimum current needed to cause consistent capture (depolarization) of the myocardium at given pulse widths. Pulse width is the time, in milliseconds, that the pacing stimulus is applied to the myocardium. In addition, a measurement of the sensing threshold of the heart is obtained. This is the amplitude, expressed as voltage, of the intracardiac signal and changes in that amplitude that can be sensed by the pacemaker.

Because dual chamber pacemakers are more complex, additional measurements need to be obtained to enable the physician to program the pacemaker. Specifically, the threshold of stimulation for both the ventricle and atrium, sensing thresholds for both the ventricle and atrium, the AV conduction interval, the coupling interval that causes AV block, and both the VA conduction (retrograde ventricle to atrium conduction) interval and coupling interval that causes the onset of VA block are evaluated.

Following implantation of the leads and after obtaining the EP studies necessary for programming the pacemaker, the physician connects the leads to the pulse generator and positions the pulse generator inside the pacemaker pocket. The pacemaker pocket is located in the subcutaneous space in the upper lateral chest, abdomen, or rarely, beneath the breast. Together the leads and the pulse generator (the pacemaker) can provide the heart with a pacing stimulus that is able to depolarize the myocardium when needed. This is essential to remember. Today's pacemakers pace the heart when needed, and complement the patient's intrinsic rhythm; they should not compete with it.

Types of Pacemakers

Now that we have discussed why pacemakers are implanted, how they are implanted, and briefly how they operate, we can discuss the different types of pacemakers and how they may be programmed.

Single chamber pacemakers have a single lead, but where is the lead implanted? Generally it's in the right ventricle, but not always. The lead may be positioned in the right atrium. This type of pacemaker is rarely seen today. It is used in patients with sinus node dysfunction but otherwise intact conduction systems. Single chamber pacemakers generally sense in the chamber they are implanted in, but not always. There are single chamber pacemakers that are positioned in the right ventricle but are also able to sense the atrium because of a sensing area on the ventricular lead located near the tricuspid valve.

Dual chamber pacemakers are more complex. They can pace and sense in both chambers. They can sense in both chambers, but pace in a single chamber. Also, they can sense in a single chamber, but pace in both chambers.

So how do you know what type of pacemaker you are seeing and how it's operating? You check the ICHD Code.

ICHD Pacemaker Code

In 1974 the Intersociety Commission for Heart Disease Resources adopted a pacemaker code so that despite the model of pacemaker the mode of operation would be known. This code was updated in 1981 to a five position code and is known throughout the world as the ICHD pacemaker code.

You will see variations of the ICHD pacemaker code. Especially the North American Society of Pacing and Electrophysiology (NASPE) and the British Pacing and Electrophysiology Group (BPEG) pacemaker codes. Often you will see the NASPE/BPEG Generic (NBG) pacemaker code utilized instead of the ICHD pacemaker code. Essentially, these codes all provide the same information.

ICHD Pacemaker Code

Position I tells which chambers are being paced.
V - ventricle   A - atrium
D - double, both the atrium and ventricle

Position II tells where sensing is occurring.
V - ventricle A - atrium
D - double, both the atrium and ventricle

Position III tells the pacemaker's mode of response to sensed intrinsic cardiac events.
T - triggered   I - inhibited D - double, both triggered
and inhibited   O - no response

Position IV describes noninvasive programmable features that vary with manufacturer.
P - simple programmable   M - multiprogrammable
R - rate modulation   C - communicating   O - none

Position V describes antitachyarrhythmia functions.
B - burst   N - normal rate competition   S - scanning
E -external control (activated by magnet or radio frequency)

The information provided by positions I, II, and III allows you to basically determine how the pacemaker is functioning. Programmable features and antitachyarrythmia functions, while fascinating, are not common and vary with the pacemaker manufacturer and model. Without the pacemaker's specifications, interpretation of these features is difficult, if not impossible. Unless you're really ambitious leave this task for the cardiologists.

Chapter 2

Pacemaker Functioning

Pacemaker Spike

A pacemaker supplied stimulus is viewed on the EKG or rhythm strip as a vertical spike.

Capture

Next it is essential to determine if the pacemaker stimulus has caused depolarization of the myocardium. In other words, is there capture? Is there cardiac muscle contraction?

Ventricular Capture

Recognizing ventricular capture is easy. Paced ventricular beats look like PVCs originating in the right ventricle (RV). The ventricular lead is positioned at the apex. To verify ventricular capture, look for a spike followed by a wide QRS, usually greater than 120 msecs. When evaluating a pacemaker patient's EKG, keep in mind that ischemic and injured areas of the heart will affect the configuration of the paced complexes. Intrinsic conduction defects will also affect the configuration of paced complexes. Positive or negative deflection of the QRS following a ventricular spike is not that important. What is important is the width of the QRS complex. It should be wide, usually greater than 120 msecs. If you are still in doubt that there is ventricular capture, take your patient's apical pulse. If he should be pacing at 70 BPM and his apical pulse is 40 BPM it's time to call the cardiologist because capture is inadequate. Pulse rates above the programmed standby rate are OK. This will be explained in depth later.

The following strip displays ventricular pacing, VVI at 80 BPM, with good capture, note the wide QRS. This patient is completely pacemaker dependent as evidenced by the absense of any intrinsic atrial ventricular activity.

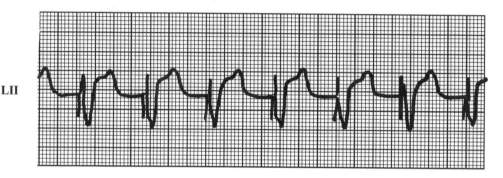

LII

As you can imagine, loss of capture for this patient is a life-threatening event and would require immediate ACLS and transcutaneous pacing until a temporary transvenous pacemaker could be inserted. Waste no time in notifying the cardiologist under these circumstances.

Atrial Capture

Evaluating atrial capture is more difficult because the amplitude of atrial depolarization is much smaller and therefore less visible on EKG than ventricular depolarization. Remember the difference in heights of an intrinsic P-wave and QRS. To observe atrial capture you may have to view several leads. Leads V_1, V_2, and lead II are best. Look for the paced P-wave or hump sign following the atrial spike to verify atrial capture; you may need a magnifying glass.

Observe the following strip of a DDD pacemaker. Note the atrial spike, the first spike from the left, followed by an odd P-wave. This is the hump sign and it verifies atrial capture. The second spike is the ventricular spike followed by the presence of a wide QRS which verifies ventricular capture.

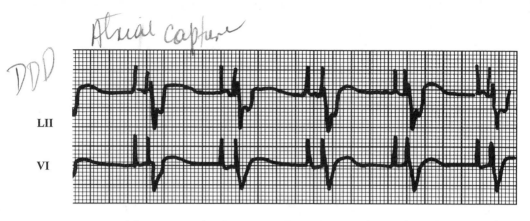

Note this next strip from a DDD pacemaker. See the paced P-wave or hump sign after the atrial spike? Compare this paced atrial depolarization to the paced atrial depolarization on the former strip. As you can see, the configuration of paced atrial depolarizations vary from patient to patient as does the configuration of paced ventricular beats.

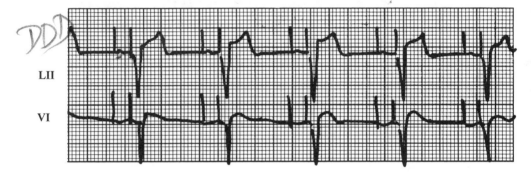

It is helpful to compare the patient's intrinsic atrial and ventricular depolarizations to his paced atrial and ventricular depolarizations to verify capture. If the patient's paced P-waves and paced QRS complexes are identical to his intrinsic P-waves and QRS complexes there probably isn't capture. Again, take your patient's apical pulse if you're in doubt. If he is supposed to be pacing at 70 BPM and his apical rate is 40 BPM capture is inadequate and it's time to call the cardiologist.

Loss of Capture

Loss of capture is the presence of pacemaker spikes not followed by QRS complexes (with a ventricular electrode) or by P- waves (if the pacemaker uses an atrial electrode). Observe the EKG strip below of a VVI pacemaker delivering a pacemaker stimulus at 80 BPM with frequent episodes of loss of capture. This patient's hemodynamic condition is threatened as a result of no ventricular depolarization and lack of intrinsic rhythm.

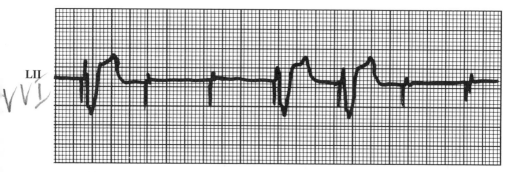

Loss of atrial capture is a potential problem for patients with dual chamber pacemakers. Failure to depolarize the atrium increases the likelihood of pacemaker induced retrograde ventricle to atrium conduction, VA conduction. As will be discussed later, retrograde VA conduction may cause pacemaker mediated tachycardia.

Notice on the following strip how the loss of atrial capture causes retrograde VA conduction which triggers rapid ventricular pacing. The retrograde P-wave is invisible to the eye because it is hidden in the downslope of the T-wave, however it is sensed by this dual chamber pacemaker and a pacemaker mediated tachycardia ensues.

Loss of Capture

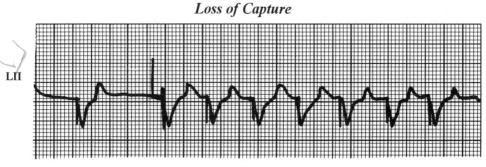

Fusion Beats

Frequently you will see paced atrial or ventricular beats that are bizarre in appearance. A combination of the patient's intrinsic depolarization and their paced depolarizations. These beats are fusion beats and they occur when the atrium or ventricle depolarize simultaneously with a paced output. This poses no problem for the patient and is therefore considered normal pacemaker functioning.

On this strip observe the intrinsic and paced fusion beats. The first three paced QRS from the left are fusion beats. The last three are strictly paced QRSs. Notice the differences in the shapes and widths of the fusion and strictly paced QRS complexes.

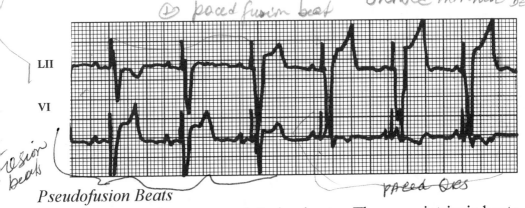

Showed intrinsic bea
① paced fusion beat
LII
VI
fusion beats
paced Qrs

Pseudofusion Beats

You may also see pseudofusion beats. These are intrinsic beats that occur simultaneously with a paced output but are unchanged by the presence of the paced output. There is no capture. The lack of capture here is considered normal pacemaker functioning. Because the intrinsic rhythm causes atrial or ventricular depolarization there is no opportunity for the pacemaker to depolarize the myocardium. The myocardium is in its absolute refractory period and capture is not possible.

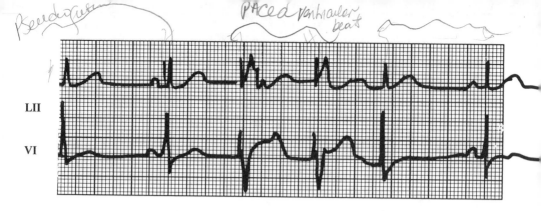

Beedique *PACed ventricular beat*

LII

VI

On this strip the first QRS after the ventricular pacemaker spike is a pseudofusion beat. It is identical to the intrinsic QRSs the first, fifth, and sixth QRSs. The third and fourth QRSs are paced ventricular beats with good capture.

Magnet Mode - VOO, AOO, or DOO

Often after the insertion of a pacemaker, the physician will request an EKG with and without a magnet. When a magnet, either a donut magnet or a horseshoe type, is positioned correctly over the pacemaker generator the pacemaker will be converted to asynchronous operation (deactivate the sensing mechanism and pace at a preset rate independent of the intrinsic rhythm). This enables evaluation of atrial or ventricular capture and can be useful in diagnosing oversensing by disabling all sensing function. Also, the magnet mode provides information about battery life in many pacemakers.

The following strip demonstrates a DDD pacemaker functioning in its magnet mode, DOO. Remember with DOO, the O in the second position means there is no sensing occurring in either the atrium or ventricle. The O in the third position means there is no inhibition or triggering in response to intrinsic cardiac events.

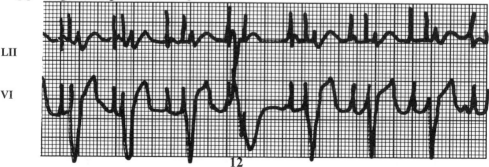

LII

VI

Observe that with this particular pacemaker model the rate and AV delay change when the pacemaker is functioning in its magnet mode for the first three atrial and ventricular paced outputs. Specifically, the pacemaker is pacing at 100 BPM and its AV delay is 100 msecs for the first three cycles. The fourth and subsequent paced outputs, while still DOO, have an AV delay of 180 msecs and pacing rate of 85 BPM. As the battery life decays, the magnet rate decreases. Plotting this rate on periodic checkups is a valuable way of detecting impending battery failure.

Note the atrial spike followed by the hump sign and the ventricular spike followed by the wide QRS. Adequate capture by both the atrium and ventricle is seen here.

LII

VI

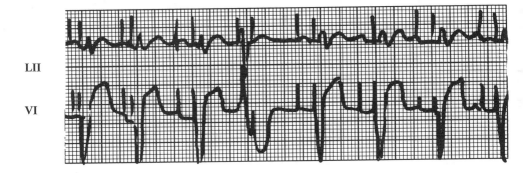

As you can see from the fifth atrial and ventricular outputs, there will be no capture if a pacemaker output is delivered during the absolute refractory period of the myocardium depolarization - repolarization cycle.

Sensing

Besides pacing the heart, today's pacemakers are able to sense intrinsic cardiac events (atrial and or ventricular depolarization). Appropriate sensing is essential to prevent competition with the intrinsic heart rhythm and in triggering of the pacemaker. Proper sensing is observed on an EKG or rhythm strip if the pacemaker is triggered or inhibited by intrinsic events in accordance with its program.

On the following strip from a DDD pacemaker, view the PVC and note how the pacemaker senses this intrinsic ventricular event and correctly inhibits ventricular pacing. Remember pacemakers should not compete with intrinsic heart rhythms.

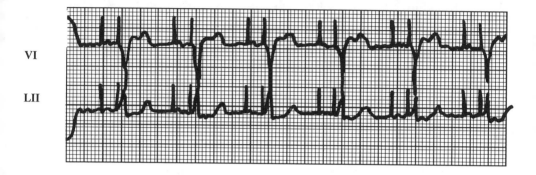

Improper sensing is either undersensing or oversensing.

Undersensing

Recognizing undersensing is simple. If the pacemaker fails to sense an intrinsic cardiac event and delivers a pacing stimulus when it shouldn't, the pacemaker is undersensing. The problem with undersensing is that the pacemaker may deliver a pacing stimulus during an intrinsic cardiac cycle that could produce a dysrhythmia. For example, a ventricular pacemaker stimulus delivered during the relative refractory period of a ventricular depolarization - repolarization cycle is essentially an R on T and could potentiate ventricular tachycardia.

Undersensing is demonstrated on the next strip when a VVI pacemaker delivers paced outputs despite the presence of a sinus rhythm. Ventricular pacing should be inhibited by the presence of the intrinsic rhythm if the pacemaker is sensing properly. The fourth paced output from the left is an R on T and ultimately the patient develops a salvo of PVCs. The myocardium is probably irritable because the pacemaker is competing with the intrinsic rhythm and stimulating the myocardium when it shouldn't be.

This can be a big problem for the patient. Notify the cardiologist as soon as possible. Night shift could wait until morning if the patient is hemodynamically stable. Certainly this patient is not because of the V-tach, and the cardiologist needs to be notified, even at 3 AM.

Oversensing

Oversensing occurs when the pacemaker senses something as an intrinsic cardiac event that is neither atrial nor ventricular depolarization. The problem with oversensing is that the pacemaker may be inappropriately triggered or inhibited. Often myocardial myopotentials; crosstalk, which is the detection of paced atrial output by the ventricular lead; skeletal muscle activity; or other artifact are mistakenly interpreted by the pacemaker as intrinsic atrial or ventricular depolarizations. Oversensing with inappropriate inhibition of pacing is a problem for the pacemaker dependent patient, because if pacing is inhibited frequently, a significant decrease in heart rate could occur.

The following strip from a dual chamber pacemaker demonstrates oversensing. Here ventricular pacing is being inappropriately inhibited by electrical activity it interprets as intrinsic ventricular depolarization. The ventricular lead senses the pacemaker's output to the atrium and incorrectly interprets the output to be intrinsic ventricular depolarization. This is termed crosstalk. Observation of the strip below confirms there are no paced ventricular depolarizations. This DDD pacemaker's ventricular lead is oversensing and ventricular pacing is being inappropriately inhibited. Fortunately, there is a ventricular escape rhythm to sustain the patient.

15

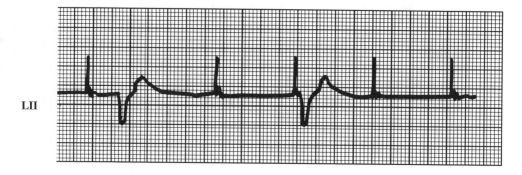

LII

Occasional oversensing may not be a problem for your patient. Again, assess your patient, if he or she is hemodynamically unstable notify the cardiologist immediately.

Another problem that results from oversensing is inappropriate pacing. On the following strip view the rather prominent U-wave between the intrinsic T- and P-waves. Then notice this dual chamber pacemaker incorrectly identifies the U-wave after the fourth intrinsic QRS as an atrial depolarization, and ventricular pacing is triggered at a rather fast rate, 94 BPM. The atrial lead of this DDD pacemaker is oversensing. It incorrectly identifies the U-wave as an atrial depolarization, and ventricular pacing is triggered.

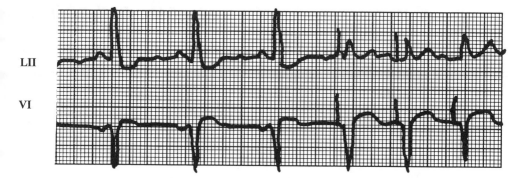

LII

VI

Again, assess your patient. Oversensing by the atrial lead with subsequent triggering of ventricular pacing at 94 BPM could jeopardize the patient's condition. Particularly if the patient has advanced coronary artery disease, congestive heart failure, or any other heart disease that may be adversely affected by rapid heart rates. Notify the cardiologist of oversensing that may be harmful to your patient.

Modes of Response to Intrinsic Cardiac Events

Inhibition

Today the most commonly implanted pacemakers are VVI pacemakers. Using the ICHD code we know this pacemaker can pace the ventricle, senses in the ventricle, and its mode of response is inhibited. The following strip shows VVI pacing at 72 BPM.

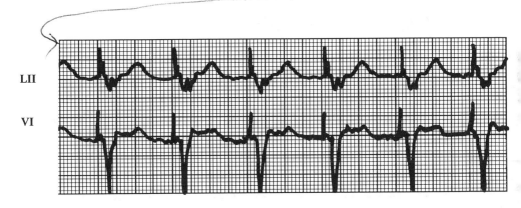

On the next strip you will notice that the patient's intrinsic rhythm interrupts VVI pacing; this is inhibition. If the patient's intrinsic heart rate exceeds the VVI pacemaker's standby rate or lower limit, pacing is inhibited. This is to prevent the pacemaker from competing with the patient's intrinsic rhythm. Again, today's pacemakers are designed to complement, not compete with patient's intrinsic rhythms. Standby rate will be discussed in depth shortly.

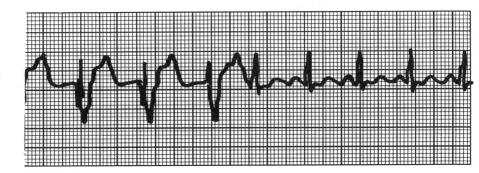

Triggered

A pacemaker may respond to intrinsic cardiac events by producing a pacemaker stimulus onto an intrinsic depolarization. This mode of response is termed triggered. Pacemakers are rarely programmed to respond to intrinsic cardiac events by triggering exclusively.

On the strip below observe the unusual appearance of the paced (fusion) beats from this VVT pacemaker. Fusion beats are a combination of intrinsic and paced depolarization. Since a VVT pacemaker triggers its ventricular output onto an intrinsic ventricular depolarization it follows that the QRSs from a VVT pacemaker are fusion beats.

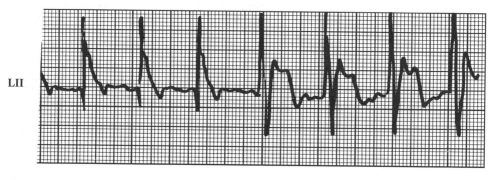

In dual chamber pacemakers, triggered also refers to the pacemaker's response to sensed atrial events. Specifically, a DDD or VDD pacemakers will trigger a paced ventricular output in response to a sensed intrinsic atrial event.

On the strip below observe the intrinsic atrial depolarization followed by ventricular pacing, this is known as atrial tracking. Again, the ventricular output is triggered by a sensed atrial event.

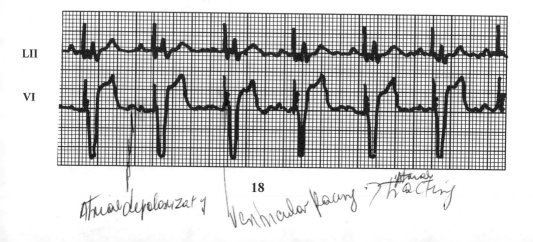

Double

A commonly implanted pacemaker is the DDD pacemaker. Again, the ICHD code tells us the pacemaker can pace both the atrium and ventricle, is sensing in both the atrium and ventricle, and its mode of response is double, both triggered and inhibited.

The following strip shows a DDD pacemaker pacing both the atrium and ventricle.

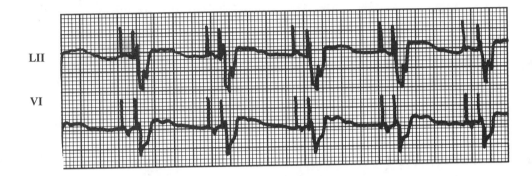

On the next strip from a DDD pacemaker observe the patient's intrinsic atrial depolarization followed by ventricular pacing. In this case the atrial lead senses the atrial activity and inhibits atrial pacing. Ventricular pacing is triggered after a set AV delay of 160 msecs. AV delay is similar to the PR interval and will be discussed thoroughly later. In other words, the pacemaker's mode of response is double, both inhibited and triggered.

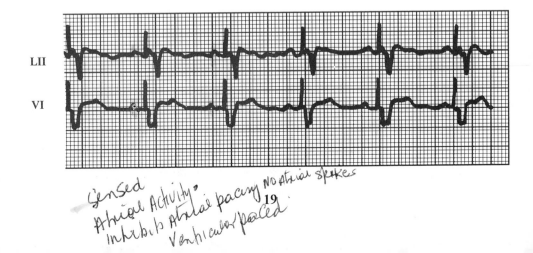

Sensed
Atrial Activity,
Inhibit Atrial pacing No Atrial spikes
Ventricular paced

On the following strip from a DDD pacemaker, atrial pacing is inhibited by the patient's intrinsic atrial depolarization and ventricular pacing is triggered. Again, this is known as atrial tracking. Atrial tracking is seen frequently and will be discussed in great detail later.

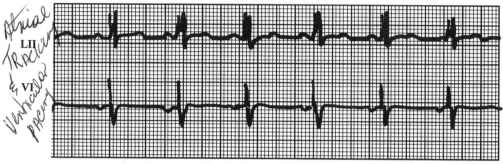

Observe the intrinsic atrial depolarization on this strip from a DDD pacemaker inhibiting atrial pacing. Ventricular pacing is triggered after a set time interval, the AV delay of 160 msecs. This is another example of atrial tracking.

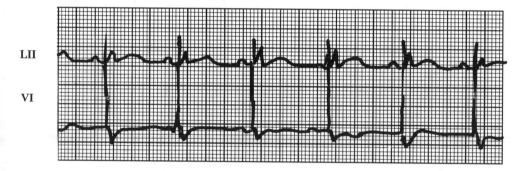

Another possibility with DDD pacemakers is atrial pacing followed by intrinsic ventricular depolarization. This is seen on the next strip.

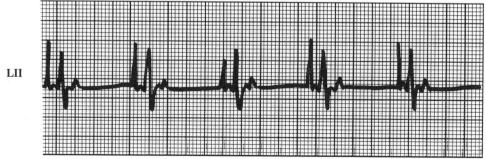

The final behavior seen in DDD pacemakers is both atrial and ventricular pacing being inhibited by the patient's intrinsic rhythm. This is seen on the following strip.

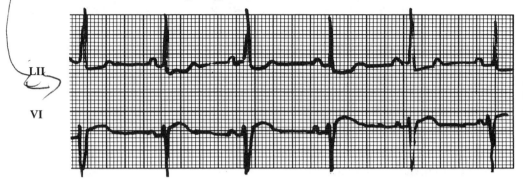

Once you know what type of pacemaker you are dealing with and how it is operating, interpreting its functioning is easy.

Standby Rate

V - V Interval

Unlike early pacemakers that simply paced the heart at a set rate regardless of the patient's intrinsic rhythm, today's pacemakers are able to sense the intrinsic rhythm and pace the heart only when needed. I can't stress enough that pacemakers complement the intrinsic rhythm, they should not compete with it.

The physician determines an appropriate minimum heart rate based upon the patient's medical condition and EP measurements obtained during pacemaker implantation. He or she then programs the pacemaker by setting the pacemaker's standby rate at the appropriate minimum heart rate. Standby rate may also be known as the pacemaker's escape interval or lower limit. Terminology varies with manufacturer and pacemaker model. Basically, if the intrinsic heart rate falls below the pacemaker's programmed standby rate pacing begins. As you can see on the following strip, as the patient's intrinsic heart rate drops below the pacemaker's standby rate of 72 BPM VVI pacing begins at 72 BPM.

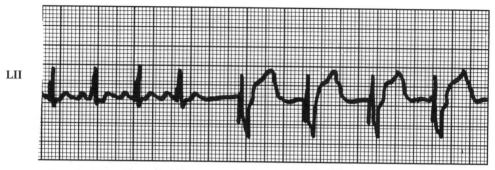

LII

In single chamber pacemakers, with the lead implanted in the ventricle, the pacemaker's standby rate or escape interval begins with a sensed intrinsic or paced ventricular event and ends with a paced ventricular event. This is the V - V interval.

Observe the V - V interval of 1500 msecs or 40 BPM on the following strip of a VVI pacemaker.

V - V Interval

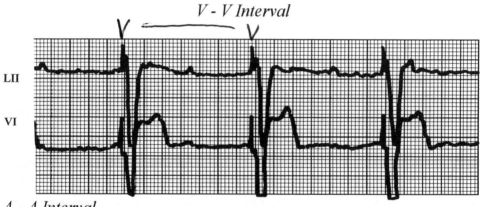

LII

VI

A - A Interval.

If the lead is positioned in the atrium, the pacemaker's preset standby rate or escape interval begins with a paced or sensed intrinsic atrial event and ends with a paced atrial event (A - A interval).

Note the A - A interval of 1000 msecs or 60 BPM.

A - A Interval

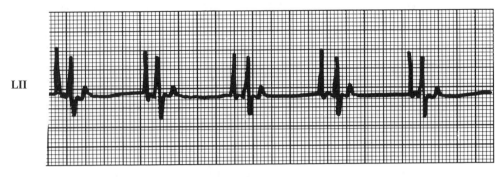

LII

Each sensed or paced event resets the timing of the standby rate. This is essential to remember.

Observe on the strip below that the paced beats after the sensed intrinsic events occur at the standby rate of 840 msecs or 72 BPM. Specifically, the distance between the second intrinsic QRS and the first paced output is 840 msecs. Also, the distance between the third intrinsic QRS and the fourth paced output is 840 msecs. Again, each sensed or paced event resets the timing of the standby rate.

840 msecs   **840 msecs**

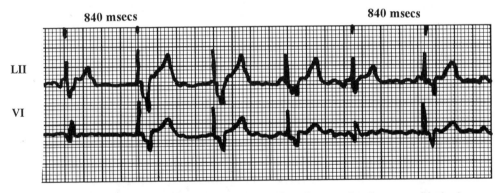

LII

VI

Observe how the PVC on the following strip from a dual chamber pacemaker resets the standby rate. The PVC occurs before the standby rate of 60 BPM(1000 msecs) and resets the timing of the standby rate. The first paced ventricular beat after the PVC is 1000 msecs or 60 BPM after the PVC. Again this is because each paced or sensed event, a sensed PVC in this case, resets the standby rate.

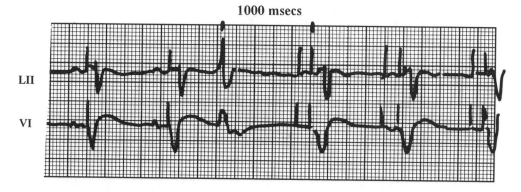

1000 msecs

LII

VI

VA + AV = V - V interval

As you can see in single chamber pacemakers, the pacemaker's standby rate or escape interval equals its lower limit. This is not the case with dual chamber pacemakers. In dual chamber pacemakers, the escape interval begins with a sensed or paced ventricular event and ends with a paced atrial even (VA interval). The standby rate or lower limit of a dual chamber pacemaker is its VA interval plus its AV delay.

AV delay is the programmed time between a paced or sensed atrial event and a paced ventricular event. An in-depth discussion on dual chamber pacemakers will be presented later.

On this strip from a DDD pacemaker observe the VA interval of 840 msecs plus the AV delay of 160 msecs equalling a standby rate of 1000 msecs or 60 BPM.

VA Interval, 840 msecs +
AV delay, 160 msecs = V - V Interval, 1000 msecs

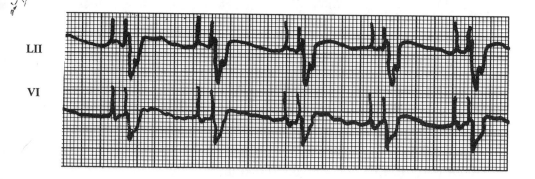

LII

VI

24

Observe on the following strip how the intrinsic rhythm inhibits VVI pacing as the intrinsic heart rate exceeds the pacemaker's standby rate of 72 BPM.

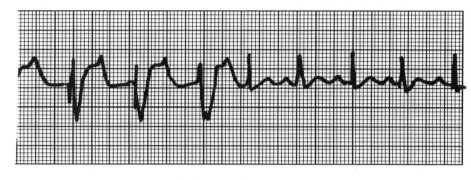

LII

Hysteresis

In reviewing EKGs or rhythm strips, the nurse may observe that the initial pacemaker standby rate is longer(or lower) than the succeeding pacing rate. Simply stated, you may observe that the standby rate from the last intrinsic event to the first paced event is longer (slower) than successive pacing. This is due to hysteresis, a programmable feature of many pacemakers. The advantage of hystersis is that it may allow the intrinsic rhythm to reoccur spontaneously, thereby maintaining intrinsic AV synchrony and decreasing pacing time, which increases battery longevity. Also, hysteresis may prevent pacemaker induced VA conduction (retrograde conduction from the ventricle to the atrium).

On this strip note the longer V - V interval, 1200 msecs, between the last intrinsic QRS and the first paced QRS than between paced V - V intervals which are 860 msecs. This is hysteresis.

Hysteresis Interval, 1200 msecs
V - V Interval, 860 msec

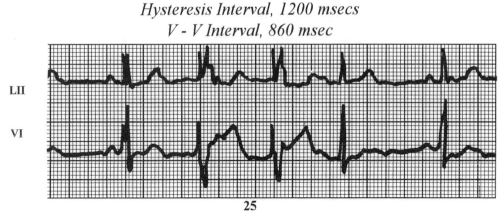

LII

VI

As you can see with hysteresis, the standby rate or lower heart rate limit is not the same as the pacing rate. On the former strip the standby rate is 1200 msecs or 50 BPM, yet this VVI pacemaker paces the ventricle at 70 BPM(860 msecs). Again this is normal pacemaker function for this VVI pacemaker with hysteresis. Also note on the former strip, that the first paced beat from the left is a pseudofusion beat. In addition, use your calibers and map out the intrinsic P-waves. Notice the intrinsic P-waves continue to occur at just under 50 BPM despite ventricular pacing. As this is a VVI pacemaker, and the ICHD code informs us sensing occurs in the ventricle only, this is normal VVI pacemaker functioning.

To briefly review the information presented thus far, pacemakers are implanted and designed to complement the patient's intrinsic heart rhythm. The pacemaker may sense the patient's intrinsic rhythm and will deliver a paced output to the myocardium when needed. Basically, pacing occurs when the patient's intrinsic heart rate falls below the pacemaker's programmed standby rate. With dual chamber pacemakers pacing will also occur if the patient's intrinsic PR interval is longer than the programmed AV delay. This will be discussed in depth shortly. Sensing and pacing may occur in the atrium, ventricle, or both. The ICHD Code informs us where pacing is occurring, where sensing is occurring, and how the pacemaker will respond to intrinsic cardiac events.

Pacemaker outputs are seen on an EKG or rhythm strip as a vertical spike. Depolarization of the atrium by a pacemaker output is verified by the hump sign after the atrial spike. A wide QRS after the ventricular spikes confirms ventricular capture. Fusion and pseudofusion beats are seen frequently and are considered normal pacemaker functioning. Hysteresis, a programmable feature of many pacemakers, allows for spontaneous return of the patient's intrinsic ryhthm. With hysteresis the standby rate that initiates pacing is slower than the actual pacing rate.

With the information presented thus far the nurse is able to interpret single chamber pacemaker functioning from an EKG or rhythm strip. If any of the information presented so far is not clear, please review the material. Adequate understanding of this information is essential before we can discuss in depth the complex, challenging, and exciting dual chamber pacemakers.

To help review the principles of pacemaker functioning, here are three strips from single chamber pacemakers. Note the patient's intrinsic rythm. Practice recognizing pacemaker spikes, identifying in which chamber pacing is occurring, where sensing is occurring, and verifying capture. Also, practice identifying the pacemaker's standby rate and recognizing hysteresis. In addition, use the ICHD code to name the pacemaker's mode of operation. Watch for undersensing and oversensing. In addition, observe fusion and pseudofusion beats.

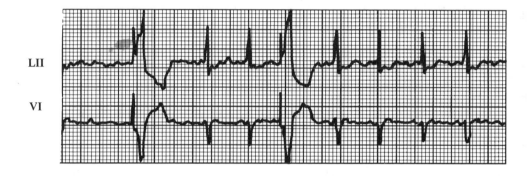

On the strip above can you identify the patient's intrinsic rhythm? It is A-flutter with variable ventricular conduction. There are two pacemaker spikes on the strip, are they ventricular or atrial? Because of the wide QRS that follows the spike we know these are ventricular spikes with adequate capture. What is the standby rate? The distance from the second intrinsic QRS and the first pacemaker spike is 840 msecs or 72 BPM. But the distance between the fourth intrinsic QRS and the second pacemaker spike is 360 msecs, not 840 msecs. How can we determine the standby rate? If you use your calibers you will note that the distance between the third intrinsic QRS and the second pacemaker spike is 840 msecs. The pacemaker simply did not see the fourth intrinsic QRS, the pacemaker is undersensing intermittently. Therefore, the standby rate is 840 msecs or 72 BPM.

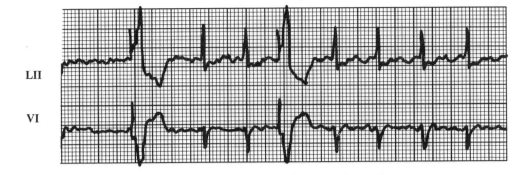

LII

VI

Is there hysteresis? We don't know. Why, because we need two consecutive pacemaker spikes to measure the V - V interval and determine the pacing rate. Once we know the pacing rate, we would compare the pacing rate to the standby rate. If the standby rate is slower than the pacing V - V intervals there is hysteresis. There are no fusion or pseudofusion beats seen here. What type of pacemaker is this? It's a VVI. Why? We've already determined it's pacing in the ventricle, V, sensing in the ventricle, V, and pacing is being inhibited, I, by the intrinsic A-flutter when it exceeds the pacemaker's standby rate of 72 BPM. Our conclusion then is that this is a VVI pacemaker, with a standby rate of 72 BPM, and intermittent undersensing. The significance of the undersensing for this patient is minimal because the patient has a hemodynamically stable intrinsic rhythm and the undersensing does not appear to be causing any instability in this patient. Therefore, we would notify the cardiologist of our findings during business hours. This does not warrant a call at 3 AM.

Below is a strip from a single chamber pacemaker.

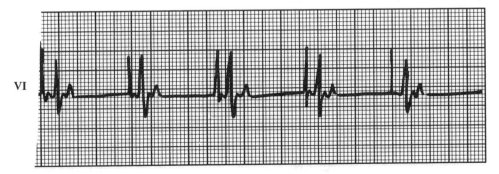

VI

LII

Can you identify the patient's intrinsic rhythm? Maybe. Maybe not. Sinus bradycardia, nodal rhythm, or asystole are a few of the possibilities. Do you see pacemaker spikes? Are they atrial or ventricular? They are atrial. Observe the hump sign after the spike, not a wide QRS complex. Which chamber is sensing in this single lead pacemaker? The atrium, probably. The atrial lead senses a lack of intrinsic atrial activity and atrial pacing ensues. However, it is possible, though unlikely, this atrial pacemaker would pace the atrium regardless of intrinsic atrial activity. Again, today's pacemakers are designed to complement intrinsic rhythms. In order to complement an intrinsic rhythm the pacemaker must be able to sense the rhythm. It is safe to assume a single chamber pacemaker senses in the chamber it is pacing in. Is there capture? Yes, the hump sign after the atrial spike verifies capture. What is the standby rate? Probably 1000 msecs or 60 BPM. Is there hysteresis? We don't know. We have no intrinsic rhythm therefore, we can't determine if the standby rate is slower than the pacing rate.

All we know from this strip is that the pacing rate is 1000 msecs or 60 BPM. How can we use the ICHD Code to identify this pacemaker? Where is it pacing? Atrium, A. Where is it sensing? Probably in the atrium, A. What is its mode of response to intrinsic events? Are the atrial paced outputs triggered onto intrinsic atrial events? No. Therefore, this pacemaker's mode of response to intrinsic cardiac events is probably inhibited, I. Therefore, this is an AAI pacemaker, with a probable standby rate of 60 BPM. However, it is possible, though unlikely this is a AOO pacemaker.

View this strip from a single chamber pacemaker.

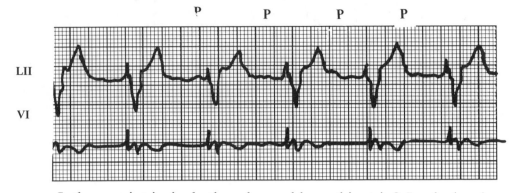

Is there an intrinsic rhythm observable on this strip? Look closely just before the third pacemaker spike. Also, note P-waves before the fourth and fifth paced beats. It appears this patient has some sinus rhythm. However none of the P-waves are followed by an intrinsic QRS and the interval between the third P-wave and the paced beat is 440 msecs. Certainly this is more than enough time for an intrinsic QRS to follow the atrial depolarization. Therefore, we can conclude that this patient's underlying intrinsic rhythm is probably a complete heart block or ventricular asystole. Which chamber is pacing? As the complexes after the pacemaker spikes are wide we know they are ventricular in origin. Which chamber is being sensed by this single chamber pacemaker? Since we have intrinsic P-waves that have no effect on the pacemaker we can assume there is no sensing occurring in the atrium. Sensing is probably occurring in the ventricle.

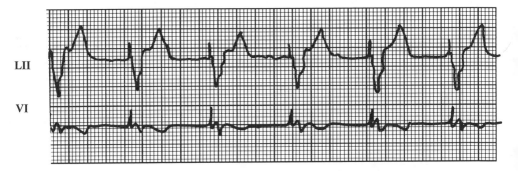

LII

VI

What is this pacemaker's standby rate? The pacing rate of this pacemaker is 70 BPM. As we see no any evidence of hysteresis, we can assume 70 BPM is the standby rate. Hysteresis would be of little use to this patient. Remember, the purpose of hysteresis is to allow the intrinsic rhythm time to resume depolarizing the heart. A patient with a complete heart block or ventricular asystole is unlikely to resume depolarizing the heart during hysteresis. Can you use the ICHD code to identify this pacemaker? What chamber is being paced? Wide QRSs after pacemaker spikes are ventricular in origin, V. Which chamber is sensing? Again, the patient's intrinsic P-waves are unnoticed by the pacemaker. Therefore, we determine that sensing is occurring in the ventricle only, V. What is the pacemaker's mode of response? Paced outputs are not triggered onto intrinsic ventricular events and there is no triggering of ventricular pacing in response to sensed atrial activity. Therefore, this pacemaker's mode of response to intrinsic cardiac events is inhibited, I. This is a VVI pacemaker with a standby rate of 70 BPM.

LII

VI

What is this patient's intrinsic rhythm? Normal sinus rhythm is seen here. Are there pacemaker spikes? Yes. Are they atrial or ventricular in origin? The wide QRS complexes after the last three spikes validate they are venticular in origin. Is there capture? The first and second QRS complexes are slightly changed by the pacemaker. They are fusion beats. No capture is achieved by the third and fourth pacemaker outputs because they are delivered during the absolute refractory period. Adequate ventricular capture is verified by the widths of the last three QRS complexes. What about sensing? Is this ventricular pacemaker sensing intrinsic ventricular events? No, it is not. Remember sensed events reset the timing of the standby rate, and we do not see that here.

We determine the pacing rate to be 72 BPM or 840 msecs by measuring the distance between the ventricular pacemaker spikes. We observe no hysteresis, so we can assume the standby rate is 72 BPM. We observe this pacemaker is not inhibited or triggered by intrinsic events. It has no mode of response to intrinsic cardiac events (it has no sensing function), 0. This pacemaker can be described using the ICHD code as a VOO pacemaker with a pacing rate of 840 msecs or 72 BPM.

Chapter 3

Dual Chamber Pacemakers

Now we will discuss dual chamber pacemakers in detail. The concepts of sensing, triggering or inhibition of pacing, capture, standby rate or escape interval, and hysteresis apply to dual chamber pacemakers as they did for single chamber devices. Except now we have to observe what's going on in two chambers simultaneously.

AV Synchrony

Dual chamber pacemakers were developed to overcome the limitations of single chamber pacemakers, mainly the loss of AV synchrony. In other words, atrial depolarization, a delay like the intrinsic PR Interval, and then ventricular depolarization. Also, the ability of the heart to increase its rate during times of physiological stress such as exercise is lost with most single chamber pacemakers. Atrial depolarization (atrial kick) is estimated to account for 10 - 30% of cardiac output and atrial kick is essential for many pacemaker recipients. For these patients AV synchrony is beneficial.

Dual chamber pacemakers differ from single chamber devices in that they mimic intrinsic AV synchrony and are able to increase their pacing rate in response to an increase in intrinsic heart rate. These are the goals of dual chamber pacing.

Observe the AV synchrony on the following two strips from dual chamber pacemakers.

On the first strip from a DDD pacemaker note the paced atrial depolarization, the AV Delay of 180 msecs, and then paced ventricular depolarization. See how the dual chamber pacemaker mimics the AV synchrony of a sinus rhythm?

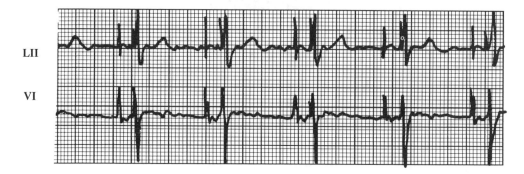

LII

VI

On the next strip from another DDD pacemaker, observe intrinsic atrial depolarization, the AV delay of 200 msecs, followed by ventricular pacing. Again, this pacemaker is mimicing the AV synchrony of a sinus rhythm. We briefly discussed this type of pacing earlier. This is atrial tracking (ventricular pacing in response to intrinsic atrial depolarization).

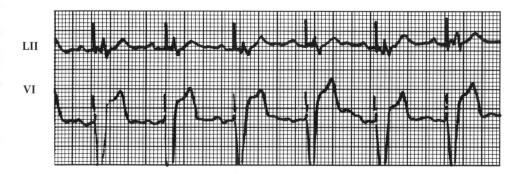

LII

VI

Dual chamber pacemakers may pace in the atrium and/or ventricle. Also, they may sense in one chamber or in both. Their mode of response to intrinsic cardiac events is triggered, inhibited, or double, both triggered and inhibited. Check the ICHD code specific to each pacemaker to evaluate what type of pacemaker you are dealing with and how it is programmed. For example, a DDD pacemaker is capable of pacing the atrium and/or ventricle, sensing in both the atrium and ventricle, and is both triggered and inhibited by intrinsic cardiac events.

The following strip is from a DDD pacemaker. Again this is atrial tracking, intrinsic atrial events inhibit atrial pacing and trigger ventricular pacing after the AV delay of 240 msecs. If an intrinsic ventricular event occurs before the end of the AV delay, 240 msecs, ventricular pacing is inhibited. Specifically, observe how the PVC occurs 120 msecs after the intrinsic P-wave and correctly inhibits ventricular pacing. Again, paced rhythms should not compete with intrinsic rhythms.

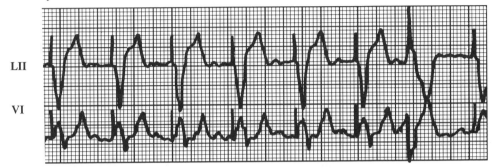

LII

VI

A DVI pacemaker, also known as an AV sequential pacemaker, can pace both the atrium and ventricle, senses in the ventricle only and its mode of response is inhibited. Remember the V in DVI informs us sensing is occurring in the ventricle only, therefore intrinsic atrial events are not sensed by this pacemaker. Note that the PVC is sensed and pacing is correctly inhibited.

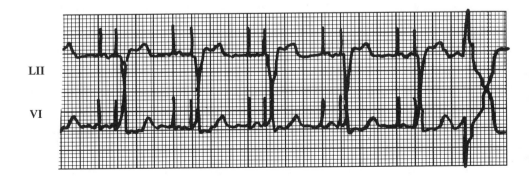

LII

VI

DVI mode is useful in patients with irregular atrial rhythms because it maintains AV synchrony by pacing the atrium and ventricle but does not track the atrium. If a patient with a DDD pacemaker converts from a sinus rhythm to A-fib or A-flutter it is desirable to reprogram the pacemaker DVI or VVI. Why? Again, a DVI pacemaker will maintain AV synchrony, but will not track the chaotic atrial activity. VVI is used almost exclusively in patients with chronic A-fib or A-flutter because atrial pacing may compete with the intrinsic atrial rhythm and percipitate additional atrial dysrhythmias. In addition, atrial capture is difficult to achieve in patients with chronic A-fib.

Observe on the following strip what happens when a patient with a DDD pacemaker converts from a normal sinus rhythm to A-fib.

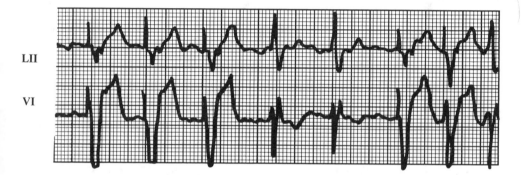

The DDD pacemaker is unable to decipher the chaotic atrial activity and maintain an AV synchronous stable heart rate. Ventricular pacing rates are often fast as the pacemaker attempts to track the fibrillating atrium. Patients with A-fib, A-flutter, MAT, or frequent PACs should be programmed DVI or VVI to prevent chaotic and rapid pacing.

How about a DOO pacemaker? It is pacing both the atrium and ventricle, is sensing in neither chamber, and does not respond in any way to intrinsic cardiac events. Basically this pacemaker is on automatic. It continues to pace both the atrium and ventricle regardless of what the intrinsic rhythm is doing. This is an antiquated pacemaker and is rarely seen today. However, as we discussed earlier when a dual chamber pacemaker is functioning in its magnet mode it is behaving DOO.

Observe on this strip of a dual chamber pacemaker programmed DOO how the pacemaker continues to pace regardless of the patient's intrinsic rhythm. Keep in mind that there may not always be capture. If a paced output falls during a myocardial absolute refractory period there will be no capture.

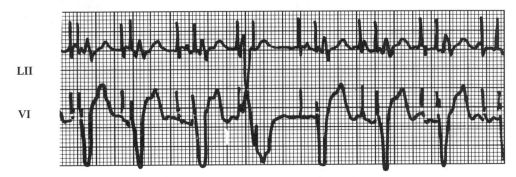

LII

VI

AV Delay

I can't stress enough that the goal of dual chamber pacing is to mimic the heart's intrinsic AV synchrony. Again, atrial depolarization followed by appropriately timed ventricular depolarization. To achieve this AV synchrony, the physician programs an appropriate AV delay.

As we discussed earlier, AV delay is the time that begins with an atrial sensed or paced event and ends with a ventricular paced event. Ventricular pacing will occur only if the intrinsic PR interval is longer than the programmed AV delay. Why? Because if an intrinsic ventricular depolarization occurs during the AV delay ventricular pacing will be inhibited. Remember pacemakers should not compete with the intrinsic rhythm.

Observe on this strip from a DDD pacemaker paced atrial depolarization for the first three cardiac events, the AV delay of 180 msecs, and then a paced ventricular depolarization. See how this mimics the AV synchrony of a sinus rhythm? Atrial depolarization (P-wave), PR interval or AV delay, and then ventricular depolarization(QRS). Also, note the maintenance of AV synchrony when the patient's intrinsic rhythm converts to sinus tachycardia.

Again, this is atrial tracking.

AV DELAY   AV DELAY

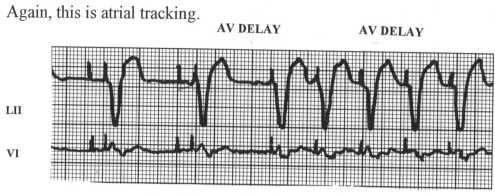

LII

VI

Rate Responsive AV Delay

At times you may see a shortened AV delay. This may be due to a rate responsive AV delay feature. When intrinsic heart rates increase, catecholamine release causes shortening of the PR interval. Pacemakers with a rate responsive AV delay mimic this behavior. The purpose is to allow atrial tracking at rapid rates. Pacemakers with rate responsive behavior, including rate responsive AV delay, are described by the ICHD pacemaker code as DDDR. The R in the fourth position informs us the pacemaker has rate modulation. You may also see this referred to as an activity mode. This will be discussed again shortly. Not all DDDR pacemakers are programmed to have a rate responsive AV delay.

Observe on the following strip that the AV delay seen is shorter, 160 msecs, than the programmed AV delay of 200 msecs. This is due to the rate response AV delay feature of this DDDR pacemaker. Also, the pacing rate is 85 BPM yet the standby rate of this DDDR pacemaker is 60 BPM. This is rate modulation or activity pacing and it will be discussed shortly.

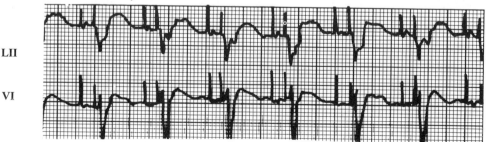

LII

VI

Ventricular Safety Pacing, VSP

Many DDD or DVI pacemakers have ventricular safety pacing (VSP) that may occur during the AV delay. VSP prevents inhibition of ventricular pacing as a result of a sensed or perceived ventricular event during the early part of the AV delay, usually during the first 110 msecs. If during the early part of the AV delay the ventricular lead senses any activity it interprets as intrinsic ventricular depolarization, ventricular pacing is triggered after a short AV delay. This is VSP. If the sensed event is a ventricular depolarization (PVC), then the paced ventricular output will be delivered during the safe part of the cardiac cycle, namely during the absolute refractory period, and capture will not occur. You wouldn't want capture here because the ventricular paced beat would be occurring on the T-wave. As we discussed earlier a paced ventricular output on a T-wave is an R on T and could potentiate a dysrhythmia.

If the sensed ventricular event is crosstalk, skeletal muscle activity or other artifact, ventricular pacing will not be inappropriately inhibited; instead the VSP will yield ventricular capture. Inappropriate inhibition of ventricular pacing is a serious problem, especially for pacemaker dependent patients because they have no intrinsic rhythm to sustain them if their pacemaker does not pace their hearts.

The AV delay seen during ventricular safety pacing varies with manufacturer and pacemaker model but is usually 110 msec. Also, keep in mind that the terminology of VSP and other pacemaker features varies with the manufacturer. Some manufacturers refer to VSP as non-physiologic AV delay.

Look for VSP on the following strip. See how the ventricular lead of this DDD pacemaker correctly senses the intrinsic ventricular depolarizations (the last two QRSs) and delivers a paced ventricular output during the absolute refractory period.

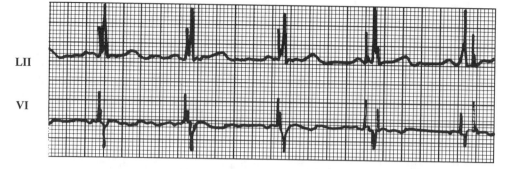

LII

VI

Can you identify the pacemaker malfunctioning seen on this strip? This DDD pacemaker should sense intrinsic atrial activity. Observe that atrial spikes are present after the last two intrinsic P-waves. Again, atrial pacing should have been inhibited by the intrinsic atrial depolarizations. The spikes after the intrinsic P-waves on the last two beats seen are obviously atrial as we can see the VSP that follows. The verdict, the atrial lead of this DDD pacemaker is occasionally undersensing.

Is it possible that the shortened AV delay seen on the previous strip is rate responsive AV delay not VSP? No. Observe the rate and circumstances of the shortened AV delay. Remember the purpose of rate responsive AV delay is to allow for rapid atrial tracking and rapid atrial tracking is not seen here. Again, atrial tracking by DDD pacemakers is ventricular pacing after a sensed intrinsic atrial depolarization.

If you see a paced ventricular event following a short AV delay (usually 110 msec) in the absence of rapid atrial tracking, suspect VSP.

Again the purpose of VSP is to prevent oversensing by the ventricular lead with inappropriate inhibition of ventricular pacing. What if the ventricular lead of a DDD pacemaker interprets crosstalk, myopotentials, skeletal muscle activity, or other artifact as ventricular depolarization and pacing is inhibited in a pacemaker dependent patient? A signficant decrease in heart rate could occur and VSP ensures this does not happen. Remember pacing should only be inhibited by atrial or ventricular depolarization, not by artifact.

To reinforce the information presented, several rhythm strips are presented and explained.

Observe the following dual chamber pacemaker rhythm strips. Note the AV delay, the patient's intrinsic PR interval, and look for safety pacing or a rate responsive AV delay. Observe the adequacy of atrial and ventricular capture. Use the ICHD pacemaker code to name the pacemaker's mode of operation.

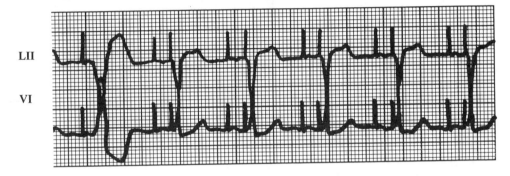

The first strip demonstrates atrial pacing with good capture, an AV delay of 200 msecs, then ventricular pacing with good capture at the standby rate of 72 BPM. How can we describe this pacemaker's mode of operation using the ICHD pacemaker code? Pacing is seen in both the atrium and ventricle, D. Because there is no intrinsic atrial activity on this strip we are not able to determine if this pacemaker can sense intrinsic atrial activity. However, we do observe this pacemaker sensing intrinsic ventricular events, the PVC, and inhibiting ventricular pacing. Therefore, we know this pacemaker senses the ventricle, V, and is inhibited, I, by intrinsic ventricular events.

This pacemaker may or may not sense in the atrium. Because we have no intrinsic atrial activity we can't determine if this pacemaker can track the atrium and trigger ventricular pacing. However it is possible. In conclusion, we observe a DVI pacemaker with a standby rate of 72 BPM and an AV delay of 200 msecs. However, as we discussed DDD is also possible.

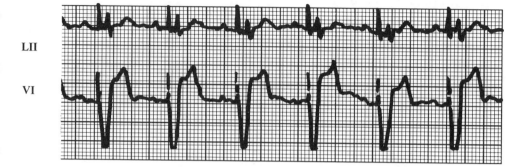

LII

VI

The second strip shows atrial tracking. Simply, atrial pacing is inhibited, I, by the intrinsic atrial depolarization. Why? Because the intrinsic atrial depolarization rate is faster than the pacemaker's standby rate. If the patient's intrinsic atrial rate is slower than the pacemaker's standby rate atrial pacing will proceed. Ventricular pacing is triggered, T, after the AV delay of 180 msecs. Again, ventricular pacing following an intrinsic atrial event is atrial tracking. Atrial tracking is in fact seen more frequently than atrial pacing preceding ventricular pacing. Remember the goal of dual chamber pacemakers is to mimic intrinsic AV synchrony. What better way is there to mimic intrinsic AV synchrony than to pace the ventricle after an intrinsic atrial event? How can we use the ICHD pacemaker code to describe this pacemaker's mode of operation? Where do we observe pacing? The ventricle, V. Where do we observe sensing, A, atrium.

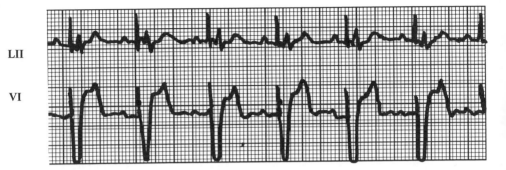

LII

VI

We have no intrinsic ventricular activity to confirm that there is sensing in the ventricle, however, we can assume there is sensing in the ventricle. Again, the purpose of pacing the heart is to complement the intrinsic rhythm and for this sensing of the ventrical is essential. Futhermore, the majority of dual chamber pacemakers are DDD or DVI. Both these pacemakers sense ventricular activity.

What is this pacemaker's mode of response to intrinsic events? Both inhibited and triggered, D, is seen here. What we see then is VAD. Is this a VAD pacemaker? Probably not. Again the most commonly seen dual chamber pacemakers seen are DDD and DVI pacemakers. DVI is not a possibility here, because DVI pacemakers do not sense the atrium. Therefore, DVI pacemakers are unable to track the atrium. Again, DDD is realistically the only pacemakers you will see tracking the atrium. It is safe to assume this is a DDD pacemaker with a standby rate less than sinus rate of 75 BPM and an AV delay of 180 msecs.

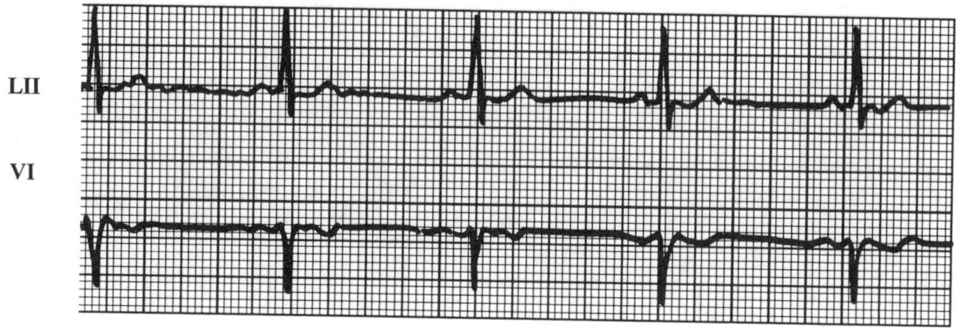

LII

VI

This strip from a patient with a dual chamber pacemaker displays the patient's sinus rhythm inhibiting, I, atrial pacing. Why? Because the intrinsic sinus rhythm is faster than the pacemaker's programmed standby rate of 50 BPM. Ventricular pacing is also inhibited, I. Why? Because the intrinsic PR interval of 140 msecs is shorter than the pacemaker's programmed AV delay of 200 msecs. Therefore, intrinsic ventricular depolarization occurs before the programmed AV delay and inhibits ventricular pacing. Remember, pacemakers should enhance the intrinsic rhythm not compete with it. No pacing is needed here because this is a stable sinus rhythm.

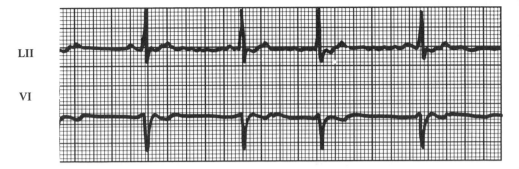

LII

VI

How can you describe this pacemaker using the ICHD pacemaker code? Where does this pacemaker pace? We see no evidence of pacing. Where does this pacemaker sense? Most pacemakers sense in the ventricle. The two most commonly seen dual chamber pacemakers are DDD and DVI, both of which sense the ventricle. We observe this dual chamber pacemaker is inhibited, I, by atrial and or ventricular intrinsic events. In reality, this is a DDD pacemaker being inhibited by a sinus rhythm. Therefore, we know this DDD pacemaker's standby rate is less than the sinus rate of 54 BPM and the programmed AV delay is longer than the intrinsic PR interval of 140 msecs. DDD is a very commonly seen pacemaker.

As you can see from the previous strips, dual chamber pacemakers are able to maintain AV synchrony by pacing both the atrium and the ventricle, by sensing an intrinsic atrial event and providing ventricular pacing (atrial tracking), and by allowing intrinsic rhythms to inhibit pacing. Another possibility is for the atrium to be paced, followed by an intrinsic ventricular beat. This is seen on the following strip from a DDD pacemaker.

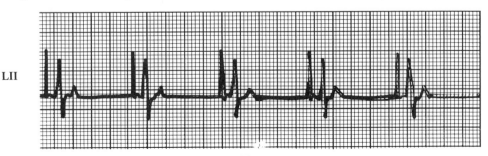

LII

To review, the DDD pacemaker's ability to sense an intrinsic atrial depolarization and to provide ventricular pacing after a programmed AV delay is known as atrial tracking. The advantage and importance of atrial tracking is that when the patient's intrinsic atrial rate increases, the paced ventricular rate also increases. This provides for maximum cardiac output during times of stress, such as during exercise. This feature of dual chamber, DDD, pacemakers has improved the quality of life for many active pacemaker recipients.

Observe on the following strip the rapid ventricular pacing in response to a sinus tachycardia.

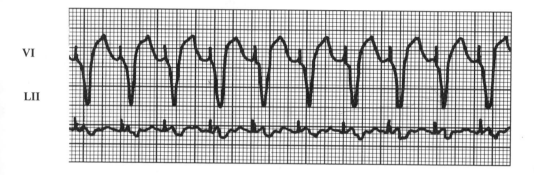

VI

LII

Rate Limiting Behaviors

While tracking rapid atrial rates maintains maximum cardiac output in times of stress, some patients are unable to tolerate rapid ventricular rates. For instance, patients with coronary artery disease or some valvular diseases could be adversely affected by rapid atrial tracking rates. To prevent rapid ventricular rates that could be detrimental to the patient, dual chamber pacemakers can limit the ventricular pacing rate. This is known as the pacemaker's upper limit or ventricular tracking limit (VTL) and is programmed by the physician.

If the patient's intrinsic atrial rate exceeds the pacemaker's programmed upper limit the pacemaker will revert to a blocking mechanism to decrease the ventricular pacing rate.

There are two main programmable rate limiting behaviors commonly seen in dual chamber pacemakers. They are Wenkebach and 2:1 or multiblock.

Post Ventricular Atrial Refractory Period, PVARP

The physician programs the post ventricular atrial refractory period (PVARP). It is this programmable refractory period that provides most dual chamber pacemakers with the ability to limit atrial tracking. The PVARP is the time following a ventricular paced or intrinsic event during which there is no atrial sensing or pacing. This programmable feature was designed to prevent DDD pacemakers from sensing retrograde atrial activity and crosstalk, but is also able to limit ventricular rates. PVARP may also be termed ventricular blanking period. As with other programmable features terminology may vary with pacemaker manufacturer. If the intrinsic atrial rate increases and the P-wave occurs during the PVARP, this atrial event will go unsensed, therefore, the AV delay will not be initiated and a new standby rate is begun with the last ventricular event.

PVARP, 325 msecs

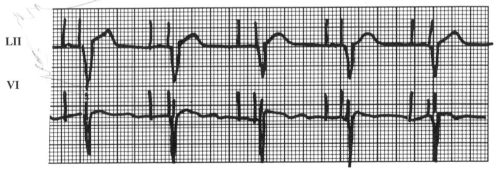

2:1 AV Block or Multiblock

2:1 AV block is usually achieved when every other intrinsic atrial event occurs during the PVARP, therefore, every other intrinsic atrial event is unsensed and ventricular pacing is not triggered. This type of VTL blocking behavior dramatically decreases the ventricular rate. Some DDD pacemakers achieve a 2:1 block at intrinsic atrial rates above the VTL by simply tracking every other intrinsic atrial event even if the atrial event occurs outside of the PVARP.

Observe on the following strips that 2:1 AV block is achieved when every other P-wave occurs during the PVARP of 360 msec.

PVARP, 360 msecs

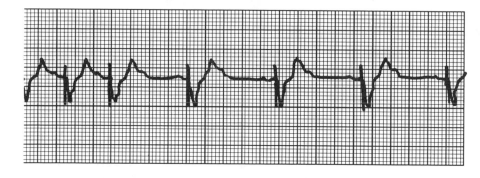

LII

If more than one intrinsic P-wave falls within the PVARP multiblock is achieved. Remember, only sensed intrinsic P-waves will trigger ventricular pacing.

Wenkebach

Wenkebach ventricular rate limiting behavior is demonstrated by some pacemakers in response to the intrinsic rhythm exceeding the VTL.

When the VTL is reached some DDD pacemakers will gradually increase the AV delay until eventually an intrinsic atrial event falls within the PVARP. The event will be unsensed and ventricular pacing will not ensue until the next atrial event, either paced or intrinsic. Observe on the following strip the Wenkebach blocking behavior of this DDD pacemaker.

AV delay in msecs

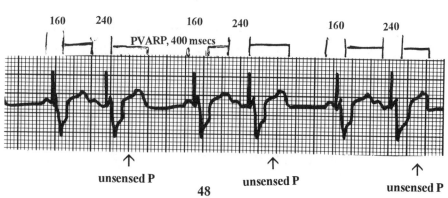

Rate Modulation

Another programmable feature of many dual chamber and some single chamber pacemakers is activity responsive pacing or rate moduluation. Occasionally, you may see a pacemaker tracking or pacing the atrium and/or ventricle above its programmed VTL. This is due to activity responsive pacing, which tracks patient activity with a piezoelectric sensor or temperature sensitive lead and computes and paces the atrium and/or ventricle at an appropriate heart rate. The purpose of this programmable feature is to maximize cardiac output during activity.

This feature permits for paced atrial and ventricular beats during the PVARP. Therefore, if you see pacing during the programmed PVARP suspect activity responsive pacing. The ICHD pacemaker codes for pacemakers with rate responsive pacing are DDDR, AAIR or VVIR. The R in the fourth position stands for rate modulation. Earlier we discussed rate responsive AV delay. It is during rate responsive pacing that you will see the shortened AV delay of rate responsive AV delay.

Observe on the following strip a DDDR pacemaker pacing above its standby rate of 60 BPM. Here pacing above the pacemaker's standby rate is in response to the patient walking. Again, this is activity responsive pacing. Activity responsive pacing may also be termed activity mode. As with most programmable features terminology varies with manufacturer.

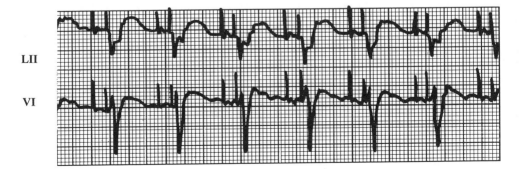

LII

VI

49

Intracardiac EKGs

Many pacemakers today have a wonderful feature to assist with pacemaker interpretation. They are able to telemetry information to the interrogator via the pacing system analyzer. The pacemaker provides a rhythm strip and denotes on the strip what the pacemaker is sensing and where it's pacing.

AS means sensed atrial event. AP means paced atrial event. VS is sensed ventricular event. VP is ventricular paced event.

Observe the strip below. Note how this intracardiac EKG informs you what the pacemaker is sensing and how it is responding. This is an exact method of pacemaker interpretation. Unfortunately, this information is not always readily available.

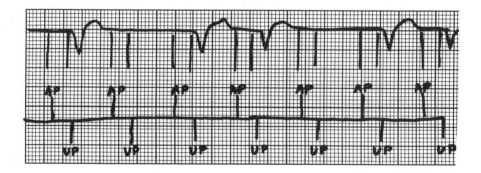

Observe on the strip above that atrial capture can not be verified. Also, there is no ventricular capture after the second and fifth ventricular spikes.

Sensing in Dual Chamber Pacemakers

As we discussed earlier, common pacemaker problems include undersensing or oversensing. If you know or are able to determine from EKGs or rhythm strips the pacemaker's standby rate, AV delay, PVARP, if there is hysteresis, VSP, and activity responsive pacing, then identifying under- or oversensing is as easy in dual chamber pacemakers as it is in single chamber pacemakers.

Undersensing

Again, undersensing is when the pacemaker fails to sense an intrinsic or paced, with dual chamber pacemakers, event. Watch for undersensing in both chambers.

Oversensing

Oversensing is when the pacemaker incorrectly identifies artifact as atrial or ventricular depolarization. Pacing may be inappropriately inhibited or triggered by oversensing. VSP prevents inappropriate inhibition of ventricular pacing by oversensing.

Here are some examples of dual chamber pacing. Look for sensing problems.

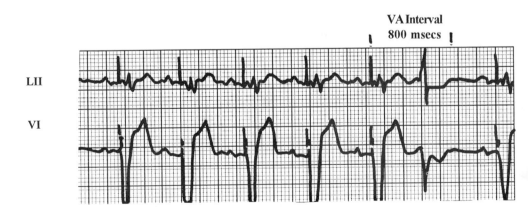

VA Interval
800 msecs

LII

VI

On the first strip the atrial lead correctly senses the intrinsic atrial events and inhibits atrial pacing while triggering ventricular pacing after the AV delay of 200 msecs. What is this called? Atrial tracking! In addition, we observe the ventricular lead senses the PVCs and resets the timing of the standby rate. Specifically, if the PVCs had not been sensed atrial pacing would have begun 800 msecs (the VA interval) after the last paced ventricular beat before the PVCs. It does not. Therefore, we know the PVCs were sensed and timing of the standby rate was reset. This is normal DDD pacemaker functioning.

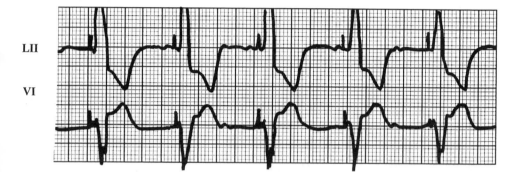

LII

VI

The above strip is indeed a challenge. At first glance this strip appears to be a VVI pacemaker pacing at 60 BPM. But a closer look in V_1 informs us otherwise. Look at the bottom of every other QRS. Notice the pacemaker spikes? These are the ventricular spikes. Note the AV delay of 110 msecs. The ventricular lead correctly senses the ventricular activity and VSP ensues or ventricular pacing is inhibited. The spikes that are causing ventricular depolarization are atrial. Can you identify the intrinsic P-waves in V_1? This pacemaker is not sensing the intrinsic P-waves. This is a DDD pacemaker whoses atrial lead is undersensing. Worse, the atrial lead is causing ventricular depolarization because the configuration after the atrial spikes is a wide QRS, not a paced P-wave.

The verdict? Undersensing by the atrial lead of this DDD pacemaker. Paced atrial outputs causing ventricular depolarization. Time to call the cardiologist. If the patient is hemodynamically stable night shift could wait until the morning to notify the cardiologist.

This next strip is from the same patient.

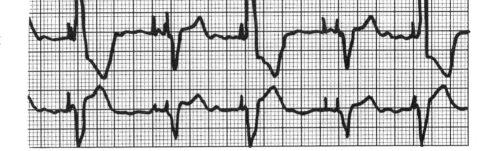

LII

VI

Notice how the second, fourth, and sixth QRS complexes look like the QRS complexes on the former strip. The presence of two spikes on this strip verifies this is a dual chamber pacemaker. Again we observe the atrial lead depolarizing the ventricle. As in the former strip, the presence of unsensed P-waves, which are well beyond the PVARP of 380 msecs verifies this DDD pacemaker's atrial lead is undersensing.

The last two strips are from a newly implanted dual chamber pacemaker. The atrial lead dislodged from the atrium and slipped through the tricuspid valve into the right ventricle. Xray confirmed the atrial lead was positioned in the upper right ventricle. This is why the atrial lead was unable to sense intrinsic atrial depolarizations and depolarized the ventricle.

Capture

Loss of Capture

Another potential problem with dual chamber pacemakers is loss of capture. Evaluate both atrial and ventricular beats to verify capture. Evaluate the following strip for atrial and ventricular capture.

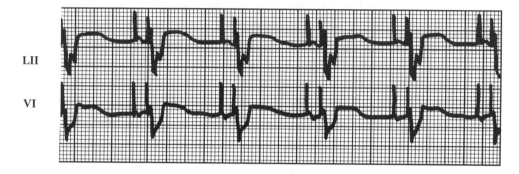

Is there atrial capture? Yes, the presence of the hump sign after the atrial spike confirms atrial capture. Is there ventricular capture? Yes, the wide QRS after the ventricular spike verifies there is ventricular capture.

Evaluate the following strip for atrial and ventricular capture.

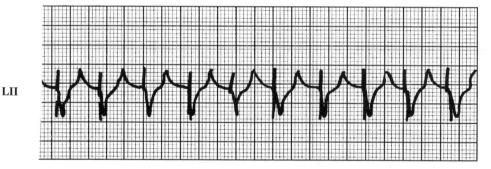

Is there capture? Atrial? No. The hump sign is absent after the atrial spike. Ventricular? Yes. The wide QRS after the ventricular spike verifies ventricular capture.

Again, the best way to confirm ventricular capture is to take your patient's apical pulse. If his paced rate is 70 BPM on the monitor and his apical pulse is 40 BPM capture is inadequate.

As mentioned earlier, loss of atrial capture increases the likelihood of retrograde VA conduction and may contribute to pacemaker mediated tachycardias as is seen on the strip above.

Pacemaker Mediated Tachycardia, PMT

A problem unique to dual chamber pacemakers is pacemaker mediated tachycardia (PMT), also known as endless loop tachycardia or pacemaker induced circus movement tachycardia. This is a rapid paced rhythm that can occur with pacemakers that track the atrium, essentially most dual chamber pacemakers.

PMT is initiated by a sensed retrograde P-wave (VA conduction). The pacemaker senses the atrial depolarization and triggers a paced ventricular beat which causes another retrograde P-wave again followed by a paced ventricular beat and a retrograde P-wave and the PMT continues.

Presently several pacemaker models are able to sense and interrupt PMT. However, it is preferable to have a long enough PVARP so retrograde P-waves are not sensed and the PMT is not initiated.

If you suspect PMT notify the cardiologist immediately because many patients are unable to tolerate the rapid PMT rates.

On the following strip observe the retrograde P-waves outside of the PVARP of 320 msecs being tracked and triggering rapid ventricular pacing after the AV delay or 200 msecs.

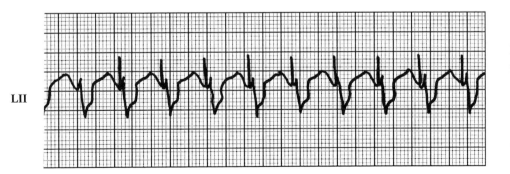

LII

Chapter 4

Nurse's Role in Pacemaker Interpretation

We have reviewed the common features of single and dual chamber pacemakers. Keep in mind that today's dual chamber pacemakers have many complex and variable programmable features. Many of which where not reviewed in this text.

The glossary at the end of the text has additional information about the complexities of pacemakers for those who are interested.

Occasionally pacemaker functioning is so complex that without the pacemaker model's specifications and intracardiac EKGs you are unable to decifer what is happening. When this occurs, it's time to call the cardiologist.

The nurse's role is to interpret common pacemaker function and to recognize pacemaker malfunctioning within reasonable limits. Anything that requires model specifications and intracardiac EKGs is maybe best left to the cardiologists.

In addition, the nurse is responsible for her patient. Any pacemaker malfunction that threatens the well being of the patient should be reported to the cardiologist.

You now have the knowledge necessary to evaluate pacemaker functioning from an EKG or rhythm strip. Using a systematic evaluation approach is helpful. To evaluate pacemaker functioning ask yourself the following questions.

PACEMAKER EVALUATION

Are there pacemaker spikes? Atrial? _____ Ventricular? _____

Is there capture? Atrial? _____ Ventricular? _____

What is the intrinsic heart rate and rhythm?_____

What is the pacemaker's standby rate?_____ Pacing rate? _____

If the pacing rate and standby rate are not equal, is there

hysteresis? _____ atrial tracking? _____

or activity responsive pacing? _____

What is the AV delay? _____ Is there VSP? _____

Is there rate responsive AV delay? _____

What is the PVARP? _____

What is the pacemaker's VTL? _____

What type of blocking mechanism does the pacemaker utilize when

the intrinsic heart rate exceeds the VTL? _____

Is there correct sensing by the atrial lead? _____

Ventricular lead?_____

If sensing is inappropriate, is there undersensing or

oversensing? _____

How can we describe what we are seeing using the ICHD pacemaker

code? _____

Let's evaluate several pacemaker strips.

LII

VI

Are there pacemaker spikes? Atrial?_____ Ventricular?_____

Is there capture? Atrial?_____ Ventricular?_____

What is the intrinsic heart rate and rhythm?_____

What is the pacemaker's standby rate?_____ Pacing rate?_____

If the pacing rate and standby rate are not equal, is there

hysteresis?_____ atrial tracking?_____ or activity responsive

pacing?_____

What is the AV delay?_____ Is there VSP?_____

Is there rate responsive AV delay?_____

What is the PVARP?_____

What is the pacemaker's VTL?_____

What type of blocking mechanism does the pacemaker utilize when

the intrinsic heart rate exceeds the VTL?_____

Is there correct sensing by the atrial lead?_____

Ventricular lead?_____

If sensing is inappropriate, is there undersensing or

oversensing?_____

How can we describe what we are seeing using the ICHD pacemaker

code?_____

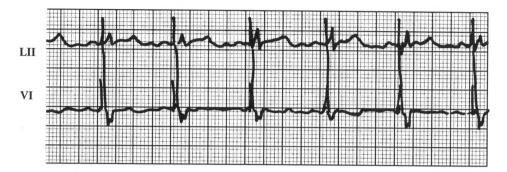

Are there pacemaker spikes? Atrial? No. Ventricular? Yes.

Is there capture? The wide QRS after the ventricular spike verifies there is capture.

What is the intrinsic heart rate and rhythm? The sinus rate is 72 BPM. Since there is no intrinsic ventricular activity on this strip we can't be sure but ventricular asystole and second or third degree heart block are possible.

What is the pacemaker's standby rate? What we see on this strip is atrial tracking with ventricular pacing at 72 BPM. We can not determine from this strip what this pacemaker's standby rate is. Remember standby rate is the V-A interval plus the AV delay with dual chamber pacemakers. We are unable to determine the V-A interval from this strip. Again, the V-A interval is the time between a sensed or paced ventricular event and a paced atrial event. We observe no paced atrial events on this strip. Therefore, the standby rate is unknown.

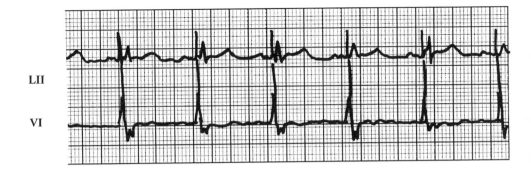

LII

VI

What is the AV delay? 160 msecs. Is there VSP? None is seen here. Rate responsive AV delay? Not seen here.

What is the PVARP? Unknown. What is the pacemaker's VTL? Unknown. What type of blocking mechanism does the pacemaker utilize when the intrinsic heart rate exceeds the VTL? As there is no blocking mechanism seen on this strip we are unable to determine the pacemaker's PVARP, VTL, or the type of blocking behavior the pacemaker utilizes to control the ventricular pacing rate when the intrinsic heart rate exceeds the VTL.

Is there correct sensing by the atrial lead? Yes. We observe the atrial lead sensing intrinsic atrial activity and inhibiting atrial pacing and triggering ventricular pacing after the AV delay or 160 msecs.

Is there correct sensing by the ventricular lead? Yes. We see no evidence of under- or oversensing by the ventricular lead. How can we describe what we are seeing using the ICHD pacemaker code? What type of pacemakers track the atrium? DDD! DDD pacemakers are able to pace both the atrium and ventricle.

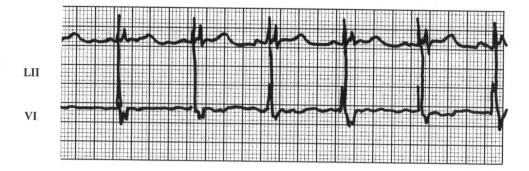

LII

VI

We don't we see atrial pacing here, why? Because the intrinsic atrial rate is faster than the pacemaker's standby rate. We see ventricular pacing after an AV delay of 160 msecs. Why? Because the intrinsic PR interval is longer than the programmed AV delay. Therefore, ventricular pacing occurs before intrinsic ventricular depolarization. Pacing in both chambers is possible here, D.

We observe sensing in the atrium and can assume there is sensing in the ventricle, D. Again, almost all pacemakers sense in the ventricle because this is neccessary to ensure the pacemaker complements and does not compete with the intrinsic rhythm.

The mode of response to intrinsic events we witness is both inhibited and triggered, D. Therefore, this is a DDD pacemaker. DDD pacemakers are realistically the only pacemakers that track the atrium. Therefore, if you observe atrial tracking, it is safe to assume you are seeing a DDD pacemaker.

LII

Are there pacemaker spikes? Atrial?_____ Ventricular?_____

Is there capture? Atrial?_____ Ventricular?_____

What is the intrinsic heart rate and rhythm?_____

What is the pacemaker's standby rate?_____ Pacing rate?_____

If the pacing rate and standby rate are not equal, is there

hysteresis?_____

atrial tracking_____

or activity responsive pacing?_____

What is the AV delay?_____ Is there VSP?_____

Is there rate responsive AV delay?_____

What is the PVARP?_____

What is the pacemaker's VTL?_____

What type of blocking mechanism does the pacemaker utilize when

the intrinsic heart rate exceeds the VTL?_____

Is there correct sensing by the atrial lead?_____

Ventricular lead?_____

If sensing is inappropriate, is there undersensing or

oversensing? _____

How can we describe what we are seeing using the ICHD pacemaker

code?_____

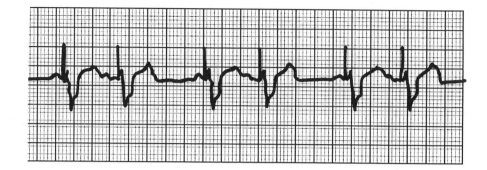

LII

Are there pacemaker spikes? Atrial? No. We see intrinsic P-waves. Ventricular? Yes. The wide QRS after the spikes verifies the pacemaker spikes are ventricular and that there is capture.

The intrinsic atrial rate is 115 BPM. As we see no evidence of intrinsic ventricular activity the intrinsic rhythm is not determinable.

What is the pacemaker's standby rate? As explained on the previous strip, a dual chamber pacemaker's standby rate can not be determined when the pacemaker is tracking the atrium. Review determining standby rate in dual chamber pacemakers in the text or the previous strip if this is unclear.

What is the AV delay? We observe an AV delay of 140 msecs, 200 msecs, and a P-wave that does not trigger ventricular pacing.
Why are there P-waves that do not trigger ventricular pacing? They are unsensed by this pacemaker because they fall within the PVARP.

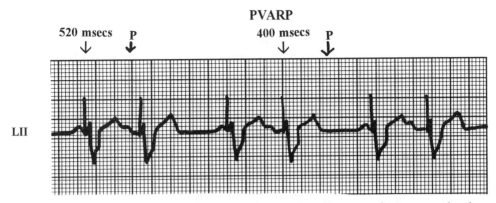

If you measure with your calibers the distance between the last sensed P-wave and the preceeding ventricular output you will determine that the P-wave is sensed at 520 msecs. However, when you measure the distance between the unsensed P-wave and the preceeding paced ventricular output you will observe it is 400 msecs. The PVARP then is between 520 msecs and 400 msecs.

What type of blocking mechanism does this pacemaker utilize to limit the atrial tracking rate? Wenkebach is seen here. This pacemaker is programmed to limit the atrial tracking rate at the VTL by gradually lengthening the AV delay. Eventually intrinsic P-waves fall within the PVARP and are unsensed by the pacemaker. Therefore, no ventricular pacing is triggered.

As we are witnessing the Wenkebach blocking behavior and the atrial rate is 115 BPM we know the VTL is less than 115 BPM.

Is there correct sensing by the atrial lead. Yes.

The atrial lead senses the intrinsic atrial rate and inhibits atrial pacing. Also, it triggers ventricular pacing after the AV delay. Furthermore, it recognizes the intrinsic rhythm has exceeded the VTL and initiates the Wenkebach rate limiting behavior.

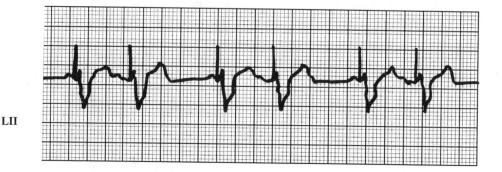

LII

Is there correct sensing by the ventricular lead? Yes. No evidence of ventricular under- or oversensing is seen here. How can we describe what we are seeing using the ICHD pacemaker code? Again, what type of pacemaker tracks the atrium? DDD!

LII

VI

Are there pacemaker spikes? Atrial?_____ Ventricular?_____

Is there capture? Atrial?_____ Ventricular?_____

What is the intrinsic heart rate and rhythm?_____

What is the pacemaker's standby rate?_____ Pacing rate?_____

If the pacing rate and standby rate are not equal, is there

hysteresis? _____

atrial tracking? _____

or activity responsive pacing? _____

What is the AV delay? _____ Is there VSP? _____

Is there rate responsive AV Delay? _____

What is the PVARP? _____

What is the pacemaker's VTL? _____

What type of blocking mechanism does the pacemaker utilize when

the intrinsic heart rate exceeds the VTL? _____

Is there correct sensing by the atrial lead? _____

Ventricular lead? _____

If sensing is inappropriate is there undersensing or

oversensing? _____

How can we describe what we are seeing using the ICHD pacemaker

code? _____

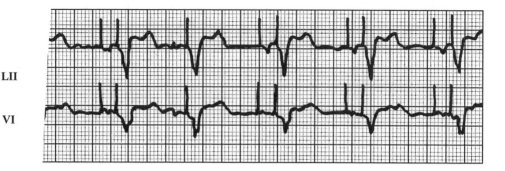

LII

VI

Are there pacemaker spikes? Yes, atrial and ventricular. Is there capture? The hump sign or paced P-wave after the atrial spike verifies atrial capture. The wide QRS after the ventricular spike verifies ventricular capture.

What is the intrinsic heart rate? As we see only one lonely intrinsic P-wave, we determine this patient has an unstable intrinsic heart rate and rhythm. Asystole, sinus brady, first, second, or third degree AV block are all possible.

What is the pacemaker's standby rate? The VA interval is 820 msecs. The AV delay is 180 msecs. Therefore, the standby rate is 1000 msecs or 60 BPM. Again, the standby rate of dual chamber pacemakers is the VA interval plus the AV delay.

What is the PVARP? Unknown.

What is the pacemaker's VTL? Unknown. Do we need to concern ourselves with VTL with this patient? No. This patient is pacemaker dependent. The third paced beat is initiated by a sensed intrinsic atrial contraction. He does not have an atrial (sinus) rhythm for the pacemaker to track.

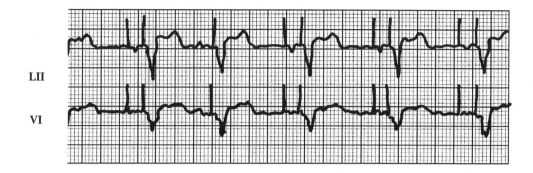

LII

VI

What type of blocking mechanism does the pacemaker utilize when the intrinsic heart rate exceeds the VTL? Unknown and unlikely that this patient would have an intrinsic rhythm that would exceed the VTL.

Is there correct sensing? Yes. We observe the atrial lead correctly sensing the lone intrinsic P-wave and inhibiting atrial pacing and triggering ventricular pacing. Therefore, we know the atrial lead is sensing correctly. We observe no under or oversensing by the ventricular lead.

How can we describe this pacemaker using the ICHD pacemaker code? Where do we observe pacing? Atrium and ventricle, D. Where is this pacemaker sensing? Atrium and ventricle, D. The pacemaker's mode of response to intrinsic cardiac events? We observe the pacemaker being inhibited by the intrinsic P-wave and triggering ventricular pacing. Therefore, its mode of response is both inhibited and triggered, D. This is a DDD pacemaker.

LII

VI

Are there pacemaker spikes? Atrial?_____ Ventricular?_____

Is there capture? Atrial?_____ Ventricular?_____

What is the intrinsic heart rate and rhythm?_____

What is the pacemaker's standby rate?_____ Pacing rate?_____

If the pacing rate and the standby rate are not equal, is there

hysteresis?_____

atrial tracking?_____

or activity repsonsive pacing?_____

What is the AV delay?_____ Is there VSP?_____

Is there rate reponsive AV delay?_____

What is the PVARP?_____

What is the pacemaker's VTL?_____

What type of blocking mechanism does the pacemaker utilize when

the intrinsic heart rate exceeds the VTL?_____

Is there correct sensing by the atrial lead?_____

Ventricular lead?_____

If sensing is inappropriate, is there undersensing or

oversensing? _____

How can we describe what we are seeing using the ICHD pacemaker

code?_____

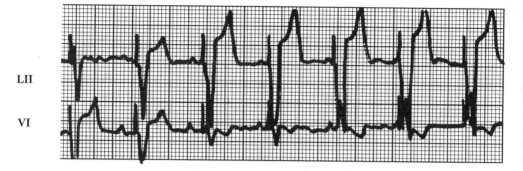

LII

VI

Are there pacemaker spikes? Yes. The wide QRS after the spike verifies they are ventricular spikes and capture is adequate.

What is the intrinsic heart rate and rhythm? We observe P-waves at 75 BPM. As the first three QRS complexes are fusion beats, a combination of paced and intrinsic QRSs, we deduce the intrinsic rhythm is probably a sinus rhythm.

What is this pacemaker's standby rate? We observe this pacemaker pacing at 78 BPM. However, because we have no completely intrinsic ventricular beats we can't be sure that 78 BPM is the standby rate. Remember, standby rate is the interval between the last intrinsic ventricular depolarization and the first paced ventricular depolarization.

What is the AV delay? Is there a consistent interval between the intrinsic P-wave and the ventricular spike? No. Is this pacemaker tracking the atrium? No. This is a single chamber ventricular pacemaker. AV delay does not apply to single chamber ventricular pacemakers.

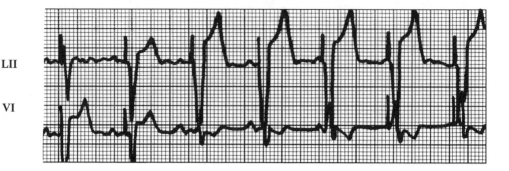

LII

VI

What is the PVARP? Not applicable to single chamber pacemakers.

What is the pacemaker's VTL? Single chamber pacemakers do not track the atrium.

Is there correct sensing by the ventricular lead? Yes, remember, fusion beats are considered normal pacemaker functioning.

How can we describe what we are seeing using the ICHD pacemaker code? Where do we observe pacing? Ventricle, V. Where do we observe sensing? We have no completely intrinsic ventricular activity to verify the pacemaker is sensing in the ventricle, however, it is safe to make this assumption. Again, most pacemakers sense in the ventricle, V. What is this pacemaker's mode of response to intrinsic activity? There is no triggering despite the presence of intrinsic P-waves and QRSs. Therefore, it is safe to assume this pacemaker's mode of response to intrinsic events is simply inhibited, I. This appears to be a VVI pacemaker with a pacing rate of 78 BPM.

I state appears to be, because in fact, this is a VVIR pacemaker with a standby rate of 60 BPM. What we are seeing is the activity responsiveness of this VVIR pacemaker. Shortly this will be clarified.

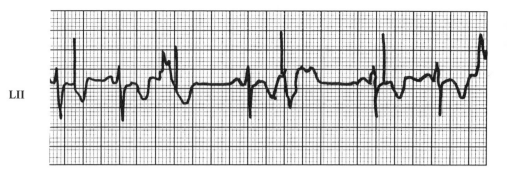

LII

Are there pacemaker spikes? Atrial?_____ Ventricular?_____
Is there capture? Atrial?_____ Ventricular?_____
What is the intrinsic heart rate and rhythm?_____
What is the pacemaker's standby rate?_____ Pacing rate?_____
If the pacing rate and standby rate are not equal, is there
hysteresis?_____ atrial tracking?_____
or activity responsive pacing?_____
What is the AV delay?_____ Is there VSP?_____
Is there rate responsive AV delay?_____
What is the PVARP?_____
What is the pacemaker's VTL?_____
What type of blocking mechanism does the pacemaker utilize when
the intrinsic heart rate exceeds the VTL?_____
Is there correct sensing by the atrial lead?_____
Ventricular lead?_____
If sensing is inappropriate is there undersensing or
oversensing? _____
How can we describe what we are seeing using the ICHD pacemaker
code?_____

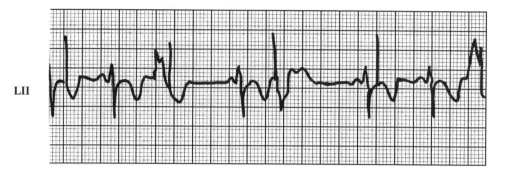

LII

Are there pacemaker spikes? Yes. Atrial? No. Ventricular? Yes. The third spike depolarizes the ventricle. The other four pacemaker spikes do not cause capture because they are delivered during the absolute refractory period of an intrinsic T-wave. Is the pacemaker tracking the atrium? No.

What is the intrinsic heart rate and rhythm? The intrinsic P-waves and QRS complexes are occurring at 80 BPM. A regular sinus rhythm with multifocal PVCs is seen here.

What is this pacemaker's standby rate? This is a good question. We see several intrinsic QRS complexes therefore, we should be able to measure the V - V (intrinsic QRS - ventricular pacemaker spike) interval and determine the standby rate. However, there is no consistent interval between the intrinsic QRS complexes and the paced ventricular outputs that follow them.

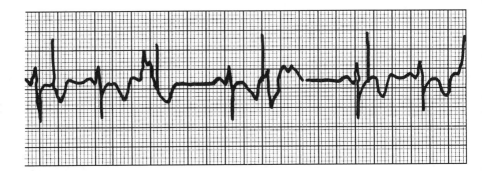

LII

We are able to measure the V - V interval between the pace-maker spikes and determine the pacing rate is 50 BPM. We observe no hysteresis or activity responsive pacing.

Atrial tracking, VSP, rate responsive AV delay, PVARP, VTL, and blocking mechanisms to control atrial tracking are not seen.

How can we describe what we are seeing using the ICHD pace-maker code? Where do we observe pacing? Ventricle, V. Where is the pacemaker sensing? This pacemaker is not sensing any intrinsic ventricular activity, O. What is this pacemaker's mode of response to intrinsic cardiac events? This pacemaker responds in no way, O, to intrinsic cardiac events. Therefore, we are seeing a VOO pacemaker.

In reality, this is a DDD pacemaker that is malfunctioning, badly. It's time to call the cardiologist. Not only is this pacemaker not functioning as it is programmed, it's also delivering ventricular paced outputs onto intrinsic T-waves. This could potentiate dysrhythmias.

The last two strips presented demonstrate that information obtained by evaluating an EKG or rhythm strip is sometimes incorrect. Or not the whole truth.

Specifically, we determined from the previous strip that we were viewing a VOO pacemaker when in fact it was a malfunctioning DDD pacemaker.

Comparing Viewed Information with Pacemaker
Programmed Parameters

What needs to be done after you've obtained the information about the pacemaker from the EKG or rhythm strip, is compare this information with the pacemaker's programmed parameters. In other words, we need to determine if the pacemaker is operating as it was programmed. As was discussed early in the text, proper pacemaker function is achieved when the pacemaker is operating as it is programmed, sensing is appropriate, and capture is adequate. There are a number of sources of information about specific pacemakers. The patient should be carrying a pacemaker identification card. The card will list the serial numbers of the pacemaker generator and lead or leads. This is a simple way to determine if the pacemaker is a single chamber or dual chamber device. If there are two lead serial numbers listed it is a dual chamber pacemaker.

The patient's chart is another source of information about the pacemaker. The cardiologist may place programming information obtained by interrogating the pacemaker on the chart.

The programmed parameters obtained by interrogating the DDD pacemaker we observed operating VOO is presented here.

Model Selected: SYNERGYST II 7070/71

Mode:	**DDD:**
Lower Rate:	60 BPM
AV Delay:	200 msecs
Upper Rate:	125 BPM
Pulse Width	
Atrial:	0.5 msecs
Ventricular:	1.0 msecs
Sensitivity:	
Atrial:	0.5 MV
Ventricular:	5.0 MV
PVARP:	325 msecs

The information above may also be written in EKG notation.

7070/71/DDD/60/200/125/325

Model

Mode

Lower
Rate

AV
Delay

Upper
Rate

PVARP

   To conclude your investigation about a specific pacemaker, you may need to refer to the manufacturer's model specifications. As previously discussed each manufacturer and pacemaker model has unique features.

   VTL blocking behaviors, antitachycardia functions, hysteresis behaviors, and PMT interruption features are a few of the behaviors you may see that may require model specifications to understand what you are viewing on the rhythm strip.

Chapter 5

Pacemaker Evaluation

The remainder of the text is devoted to having the nurse practice evaluating pacemaker function from rhythm strips. Comparing your findings with the pacemaker's programming parameters. And then assessing if the pacemaker is functioning as it is programmed. In other words, evaluating if the pacemaker is functioning normally.

A rhythm strip, programming parameters, and an explanation are provided with each strip.

We will begin by comparing the information we obtained earlier about the DDD pacemaker we viewed operating VOO with the programmed parameters for this DDD pacemaker.

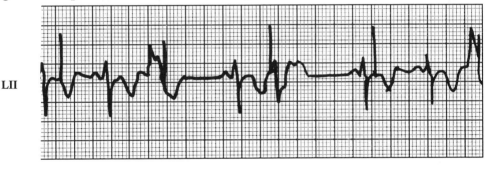

LII

	Parameters Seen on Rhythm Strip	Programmed Parameters
Mode:	VOO	DDD
Standby Rate:	50 BPM	60 BPM
Pacing Rate:	50 BPM	60 BPM
Hysteresis:	not seen	off
VTL:	not seen	125 BPM
AV Delay:	not seen	200 msecs
Rate Responsive Pacing:	not seen	off
PVARP:	not seen	325 msecs
VSP:	not seen	on

79

Does what we observe on the rhythm strip agree with the programmed parameters? No. The verdict? This DDD pacemaker is operating VOO. It's time to call the cardiologist.

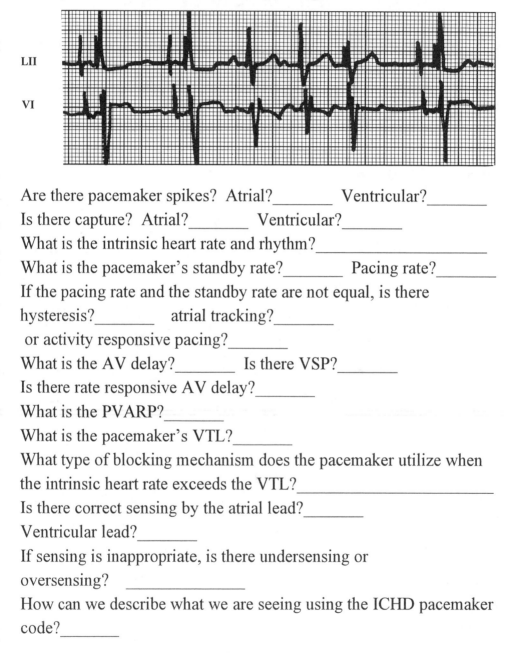

Are there pacemaker spikes? Atrial?_____ Ventricular?_____

Is there capture? Atrial?_____ Ventricular?_____

What is the intrinsic heart rate and rhythm?_____

What is the pacemaker's standby rate?_____ Pacing rate?_____

If the pacing rate and the standby rate are not equal, is there

hysteresis?_____ atrial tracking?_____

 or activity responsive pacing?_____

What is the AV delay?_____ Is there VSP?_____

Is there rate responsive AV delay?_____

What is the PVARP?_____

What is the pacemaker's VTL?_____

What type of blocking mechanism does the pacemaker utilize when

the intrinsic heart rate exceeds the VTL?_____

Is there correct sensing by the atrial lead?_____

Ventricular lead?_____

If sensing is inappropriate, is there undersensing or

oversensing? _____

How can we describe what we are seeing using the ICHD pacemaker

code?_____

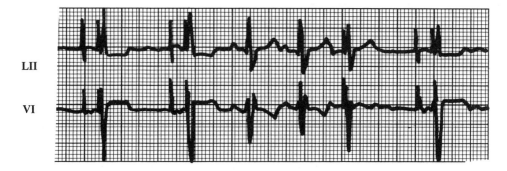

LII

VI

Atrial and ventricular pacemaker spikes are present. The hump signs after the atrial spikes verify atrial capture. The wide QRSs after the ventricular spikes verify ventricular capture.

Some intrinsic irregular sinus rhythm is seen on this strip. The V-A interval of 820 msecs plus the AV delay of 180 msecs equals a V-V interval of 1000 msecs or 60 BPM. The standby rate is 60 BPM. The pacing rate is also 60 BPM. No hysteresis is seen. We do observe atrial tracking of the third intrinsic P-waves. No VSP is seen here.

As we observe no unsensed atrial activity, we are unable to determine the PVARP, VTL, or the blocking mechanism this pacemaker utilizes to limit the VTL.

Both the atrial and ventricular lead are sensing appropriately. There are two obvious intrinsic P-waves on this strip. The third is hidden in a T-wave but is correctly sensed by the pacemaker, and ventricular pacing is triggered.

We observe pacing in both the atrium and ventricle, D. Sensing is seen in both chambers, D. We observe this pacemaker's mode of response to intrinsic cardiac events is both inhibited and triggered, D. Therefore, this appears to be a DDD pacemaker. Also, we observe this pacemaker tracking the atrium. What type of pacemakers track the atrium? DDD!

Now let's compare what we observed on the rhythm strip with this pacemaker's programmed parameters to complete our evaluation.

	Parameters Seen on Rhythm Strip	**Programmed Parameters**
Mode:	DDD	DDD
Standby Rate:	60 BPM	60 BPM
Pacing Rate:	60 BPM	60 BPM
Hysteresis:	not seen	off
VTL:	unknown	120 BPM
AV Delay:	180 msecs	180 msecs
Rate Responsive Pacing:	not seen	off
PVARP:	unknown	300 msecs
VSP:	not seen	on

Does what we observe on the rhythm strip agree with the programmed parameters? Yes it does. The verdict is a normally functioning DDD pacemaker.

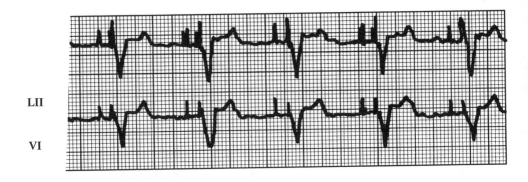

LII

VI

Are there pacemaker spikes? Atrial?_____ Ventricular?_____

Is there capture? Atrial?_____ Ventricular?_____

What is the intrinsic heart rate and rhythm?_____

What is the pacemaker's standby rate?_____ Pacing rate?_____

If the pacing rate and the standby rate are not equal, is there

hysteresis?_____ atrial tracking?_____ or activity

responsive pacing?_____

What is the AV delay?_____ Is there VSP?_____

Is there rate responsive AV delay?_____

What is the PVARP?_____

What is the pacemaker's VTL?_____

What type of blocking mechanism does the pacemaker utilize when

the intrinsic heart rate exceeds the VTL?_____

Is there correct sensing by the atrial lead?_____

Ventricular lead?_____

If sensing is inappropriate, is there undersensing or

oversensing?_____

How can we describe what we are seeing using the ICHD pacemaker

code?_____

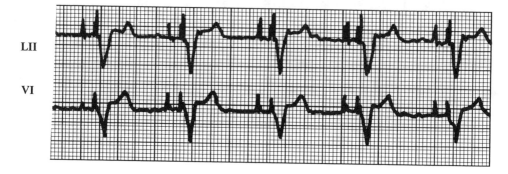

LII

VI

Atrial and ventricular spikes are seen. Deviation from the baseline following the atrial spikes is inconsistent and minute. Therefore, atrial capture can't be confirmed. Wide QRS complexes after the ventricular spikes verify ventricular capture.

Intrinsic P-waves occur at approximately 72 BPM. No intrinsic ventricular complexes are seen despite the long intervals seen after several intrinsic P-waves. This patient is pacemaker dependent because he has no intrinsic ventricular activity to sustain him in the event of pacemaker malfunction.

The pacemaker's pacing rate is 60 BPM. Hysteresis is of no use to patients without intrinsic ventricular activity. Also, there is no atrial tracking of intrinsic P-waves. Therefore, we can assume the pacing rate we observe is also the standby rate.

Activity responsive pacing is not seen.

The AV delay is 140 msecs. No VSP is seen.

We observe no triggering of pacing by intrinsic events ,therefore, we can assume this pacemaker's mode of response to sense intrinsic activity is inhibited, I. We conclude then, this is a DVI pacemaker. While not as commonly utilized as DDD pacemakers, DVI is a frequently seen dual chamber pacemaker.

Now compare what we observed on the strip with this pacemaker's programmed parameters to complete our evaluation.

	Parameters Seen on Rhythm Strip	Programmed Parameters
Mode:	DVI	DVI
Standby Rate:	60 BPM	60 BPM
Pacing Rate:	60 BPM	60 BPM
Hysteresis:	not seen	off
VTL:	not applicable	not applicable
AV Delay:	140 msecs	140 msecs
Rate Responsive Pacing:	not seen	off
PVARP:	not applicable	not applicable
VSP:	not seen	on

Does what we observe on the rhythm strip agree with the programmed parameters? Yes it does. The verdict is a DVI pacemaker with questionable atrial capture.

LII

Are there pacemaker spikes? Atrial?_____ Ventricular?_____

Is there capture? Atrial?_____ Ventricular?_____

What is the intrinsic heart rate and rhythm?_____

What is the pacemaker's standby rate?_____ Pacing
rate?_____ If the pacing rate and the standby rate are not equal,
is there
hysteresis?_____ atrial tracking?_____ or activity responsive
pacing?_____

What is the AV delay?_____ Is there VSP?_____

Is there rate responsive AV delay?_____

What is the PVARP?_____

What is the pacemaker's VTL?_____

What type of blocking mechanism does the pacemaker utilize when
the intrinsic heart rate exceeds the VTL?_____

Is there correct sensing by the atrial lead?_____
Ventricular lead?_____

If sensing is inappropriate, is there undersensing or
ovesensing? _____

How can we describe what we are seeing using the ICHD pacemaker
code?_____

86

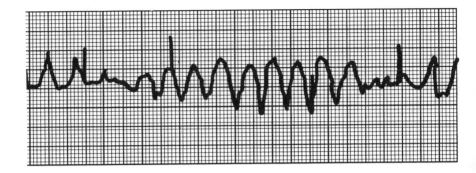

LII

Single pacemaker spikes are seen. Usually when single spikes are present, they are ventricular.

There is no capture. Consistent wide QRS complexes after the spikes are absent. The intrinsic rhythm is torsades de point.

The pacemaker's standby rate is probably 60 BPM. The V - V interval between the second and third pacemaker spikes is 1000 msecs or 60 BPM. Also, pacemaker spikes are occuring at 60 BPM between the fourth and fifth spikes.

AV delay, rate responsive AV delay, atrial tracking, VSP, PVARP, and VTL do not apply to single chamber ventricular pacemakers.

The pacemaker makes a valiant attempt to sense and interpret this chaotic ventricular rhythm. When no intrinsic ventricular depolarizations are sensed, ventricular pacing is initiated. Because we see a change in some of the V - V intervals, we know the pacemaker is occasionally sensing the chaotic intrinsic ventricular activity. When intrinsic ventricular activity is sensed, ventricular pacing is appropriately inhibited.

The potential for inappropriate sensing by the pacemaker is the least of this patient's problems.

Pacing is occurring in the ventricle only, V. Sensing is being attempted in the ventricle only, V. We observe this pacemaker being inhibited by intrinsic activity, I. The ICHD pacemaker code for this pacemaker is VVI.

Now compare what we observe on the strip with the pacemaker's programmed parameters to complete our evaluation.

	Parameters Seen on Rhythm Strip	**Programmed Parameters**
Mode:	VVI	VVI
Standby Rate:	60 BPM	60 BPM
Pacing Rate:	60 BPM	60 BPM
Hysteresis:	not seen	off
VTL:	not applicable	not applicable
AV Delay:	not applicable	not applicable
Rate Responsive Pacing:	not seen	none
PVARP:	not applicable	not applicable
VSP:	not applicable	not applicable

Does what we observe on the rhythm strip agree with the programmed parameters? Yes it does. The verdict is a normally functioning VVI pacemaker. Unfortunately, the myocardium is not functioning as well as the pacemaker. It's time to call the cardiologist. Stat!

LII

VI

Are there pacemaker spikes? Atrial?_____ Ventricular?_____

Is there capture? Atrial?_____ Ventricular?_____

What is the intrinsic heart rate and rhythm?_____

What is the pacemaker's standby rate?_____ Pacing rate?_____

If the pacing rate and standby rate are not equal, is there

hysteresis?_____ atrial tracking?_____ or activity responsive

pacing?_____

What is the AV delay?_____ Is there VSP?_____

Is there rate responsive AV delay?_____

What is the PVARP?_____

What is the pacemaker's VTL?_____

What type of blocking mechanism does the pacemaker utilize when

the intrinsic heart rate exceeds the VTL?_____

Is there correct sensing by the atrial lead?_____

Ventricular lead?_____

If sensing is inappropriate, is there undersensing or

oversensing? _____

How can we describe what we are seeing using the ICHD pacemaker

code?_____

LII

VI

Wide QRSs after the pacemaker spikes inform us the spikes are ventricular and capture is adequate.

Observed is an atrial rate of 92 BPM with a four beat run of V-tach.

The standby rate can not be determined. Standby rate is the interval between a ventricular event and a paced atrial event in dual chamber pacemakers. We observe atrial tracking at 92 BPM. What type of pacemakers track the atrium? DDD!

The AV delay is 160 msecs. No VSP or rate responsive AV delay is apparent.

We observe no blocking mechanism, therefore, we are unable to determine the VTL, PVARP, or the blocking mechanism used to limit the VTL by this pacemaker.

Both atrial and ventricular sensing is appropriate.

This pacemaker is seen pacing the ventricle, V. Sensing is seen occurring in the atrium and ventricle, D. This pacemaker's mode of response to intrinsic cardiac events is both inhibited and triggered, D. Is this a VDD pacemaker? It's possible, but not likely. What type of commonly seen pacemakers track the atrium? DDD!

Now compare what we observed on the strip with this pacemaker's programmed parameters to complete our evaluation.

	Parameters Seen on Rhythm Strip	Programmed Parameters
Mode:	VDD, more likely DDD	DDD
Standby Rate:	not determinable	50 BPM
Pacing Rate:	atrial tracking seen	50 BPM
Hysteresis:	not seen	off
VTL:	not determinable	120 BPM
AV Delay:	160 msecs	160 msecs
Rate Responsive Pacing:	not seen	off
PVARP:	not determinable	320 msecs
VSP:	not seen	on

Does what we observe on the rhythm strip agree with the programmed parameters? Yes it does. The verdict is a normally functioning DDD pacemaker.

The glossary at the end of the text has additional information about the complexities of pacemakers for those who are interested.

Occasionally pacemaker functioning is so complex that without the pacemaker model's specifications and intracardiac EKGs, you are unable to decipher what is happening. When this occurs, it's time to call the cardiologist.

The nurse's role is to interpret common pacemaker function and to recognize pacemaker malfunctioning within reasonable limits. Anything that requires model specifications and intracardiac EKGs is maybe best left to the cardiologists.

In addition, the nurse is responsible for her patient. Any pacemaker malfunction that threatens the well being of the patient should be reported to the cardiologist.

You now have the knowledge necessary to evaluate pacemaker functioning from an EKG or rhythm strip. Happy interpreting!

Carol J.V.O. Wallace R.N.

Glossary

Activity responsive pacing - A feature of many pacemakers. The pacemaker tracks the patient's physical activity with a piezoelectric sensor or temperature sensitive lead, computes an appropriate heart rate based on activity or body temperature, and then paces at the computed rate. The rate may exceed the VTL during activity responsive pacing. The sinus node can over-ride the activity responsive pacing at any time. The purpose of activity responsive pacing is to achieve maximum cardiac output during activity or fever.

Atrial tracking - A pacing mode in which the ventricles are paced in synchrony with sensed intrinsic atrial events. Also known as AV synchronous pacing.

AV delay - The programmed time interval, expressed in milliseconds, beginning with an atrial sensed or paced event and ending with a ventricular paced event.

Battery longevity - The life of the pacemaker's lithium battery, which is its power source. Factors that affect battery life are energy output, pacing rate, pulse duration, pacing time and battery capacity. Frequently as the battery nears the end of its life, the pacemaker will pace at a rate lower than its programmed lower limit.

Bipolar lead - see Lead.

Blanking - An absolute refractory period in the sensing circuit at the time of pacemaker output or intrinsic depolarization.

Capture - The depolarization of cardiac muscle by a pacemaker output.

Crosstalk - The unwanted sensing of potentials or pacemaker outputs generated in one chamber (atrial or ventricular) and sensed by the other chamber.

Dual chamber pacemaker - see Pacemaker.

Fallback - A feature of some dual chamber pacemakers to limit the ventricular pacing rate. If the intrinsic atrial rate exceeds the pacemaker's programmed VTL, the pacemaker will gradually increase the AV delay to decrease the ventricular pacing rate to a programmed rate, the fallback rate.

Fusion beat - A depolarization that is produced by intrinsic and paced depolarizations occurring simultaneously and has characteristics of both.

Hump sign - The hump sign or paced P-wave is a "hump" seen after the atrial spike that provides evidence of atrial capture.

Hysteresis - A programmable feature where the first pacemaker escape interval is longer that those that follow. Hysteresis is designed to allow for the spontaneous return of the intrinsic heart rhythm, preventing retrograde VA conduction and conserving battery life. The pacemaker will not begin to pace until the patient heart rate falls below a certain rate, but when the pacemaker begins pacing, it paces at a rate faster than the escape rate.

Impedence - The sum of all the resistances to energy flow to the cardiac muscle.

Inhibited - A pacemaker response to intrinsic cardiac events. If an intrinsic cardiac event is sensed during the pacemaker escape interval and AV delay with dual chamber pacemakers, the pacemaker will not produce an output. It is inhibited.

Lead - The part of the pacemaker that delivers the electrical stimulus to the cardiac muscle. The lead may be bipolar or unipolar. Bipolar leads have a cathode (-) tip and the anode (+) is located 1 - 3 cm proximal to the cathode tip on the same lead. The electric circuit is completed inside the heart and is therefore less sensitive to skeletal muscle or other artifact. With unipolar leads, the pulse generator is the anode (+) and the lead tip is the cathode (-).

Magnet mode - The pacing response of a pacemaker to the closure of its magnet switch (Reed switch). AOO, VOO, or DOO. When a magnet has been applied over the generator, the pacemaker paces in an asynchronous manner at a predetermined rate.

Oversensing - see Sensing.

Pacemaker - An implanted device that regulates heart rhythm and rate by delivering an electrical stimulus to the heart that is able to depolarize cardiac muscle when intinsic heart rhythm or rate is inadequate. The device consists of a battery/timer, also known as the pulse generator, and leads that are generally implanted in the right atrium, right ventricle, or both the right atrium and right ventricle. Single chamber pacemakers have a single lead, and dual chamber pacemakers have two leads.

Pacemaker escape interval - The programmed time interval, in milliseconds or beats per minute (BPM), between a sensed or paced event and the next paced event. Also known as the standby rate or lower limit.

Pacemaker initiated arrhythmia - An arrhythmia that is initiated by a pacemaker stimulus and continues without further pacemaker functioning.

Pacemaker mediated tachycardia (PMT) - A rapid paced rhythm which can occur with atrial tracking pacemakers. A retrograde atrial depolarization triggers a ventricular paced output which causes another retrograde atrial depolarization, and subsequent paced ventricular output and the PMT continues. PMT is also known as endless loop tachycardia or pacemaker mediated circus movement tachycardia.

Post ventricular atrial refractory period (PVARP) - The atrial refractory period following a paced ventricular event during which there is no atrial sensing or pacing. This programmable feature is designed to prevent DDD pacemakers from sensing retrograde atrial activity.

Pseudofusion beat - An intrinsic cardiac depolarization with a superimposed pacemaker spike. Unlike fusion beats, the appearance of the intrinsic depolarization is unchanged by the pacemaker output, except for the presence of the pacemaker spike.

Pulse width - The programmable duration of time, in milliseconds, the pacemaker stimulus is applied to the cardiac muscle.

Resistance (R) - The opposition to electrical current, expressed in ohm.

Safety margin - The heart's stimulation threshold x 3, in newly implanted pacemakers, or x 2 approximately six months after implantation.

Sensing - The pacemaker's ability to recognize intrinsic cardiac events because of changes in electrical activity within the myocardium. Undersensing occurs when the pacemaker fails to recognize intrinsic cardiac events. Oversensing occurs when the pacemaker interprets artifact as intrinsic cardiac events.

Single chamber pacemaker - see Pacemaker.

Stimulation threshold - The minimum current, in milliampere, when delivered in diastole after the relative and absolute refractory periods, that is able to cause consistent depolarization of the cardiac muscle.

Triggered - A pacemaker response to intrinsic cardiac events. An intrinsic cardiac event produces a pacemaker stimulus onto the intrinsic depolarization. This mode of response is rarely used alone. Usually pacemakers are programmed to respond to intrinsic cardiac events by inhibition and triggering.

Undersensing - see Sensing.

Unipolar lead - see Lead.

VA interval - The programmed time interval, in milliseconds, beginning with a paced or intrinsic ventricular event and ending with a paced atrial event.

Voltage (V) - The force causing electron movement.

REFERENCES

Akiyama, T. (1984). Ventricular Safety Pacing in DDD and DVI Pacemakers. *Medtronic News.* 9.

Baker, R., Alder, S. & Sanders, R. (1984). *Advances in Dual - Chamber Pacing, Sensing, and Telemetry.* Med Medical Electronics, reprinted from the September 1984 Issue, (Intermedics Incorporated). Angleton, TX.

Benditt, D. G., Milstein, S., Reyes, W. J. & Buetikofer, J. (1988) The Need for Rate Response in Cardiac Pacing. *Medtronic News.* 3.

Bernstein, A. D., Camm, A. J., Fletcher, R. D., Gold, R. D. Rickards, A. F., Symth, N. P., Spielman, S. R., & Sutton, R. (1987). The NASPE/ BPEG generic pacemaker code for antibradyarrhythmia and adaptive-rate pacing and antitachyarrhythmia devices. *PACE,* 10. 794-799.

Heymans, M. (1983). Karel de Dulk interviewed, DDD Pacing in the Presence of Retrograde Conduction. *Medtronic News.* 9.

Furman, S., Hayes, D. L. & Holmes, D. R.,Jr. (1986). *A Practice of Cardiac Pacing.* New York: Futura.

Hauser, R. (1981). Indications for Pacing Bradyarrhythmias. *Medtronic News.* 6.

Intermedics. (no date). *Current Trends in Cardiac Pacing.* Angleton, TX.

Intermedics. (1986). *Guide To DDD Pacing.* Angleton, TX.

Medtronic. (no date). *A Lecture Series, Dual Chamber Pacing Operations.* Minneapolis, MN.

Levine, P. A., Schuler, H. & Lingren, A. (1988). *Pacemaker ECG Utilization of Pulse Generator Telemetry - A Benefit of Space Age Technology.* Presented at Cardiostim 1988. Sweden: Seimens-Elema, AB.

Moses, H. W., Schneider, J. A., Miller, B. D. & Taylor, G. J. (1991). *A Practical Guide to Cardiac Pacing (3rd ed.).* Boston: Little, Brown and Company.

Parsonnet, V., Crawford, C. C. & Berstein, A. D. (1984). The 1981 United States Survey of Cardiac Pacing Practices. *Journal of the American College of Cardiologists.* 3, 1321.

Sutton, R. (1982). Pacing Modes. *Medtronic News.* 3.

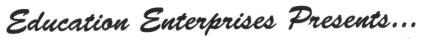

The Title Says It All...

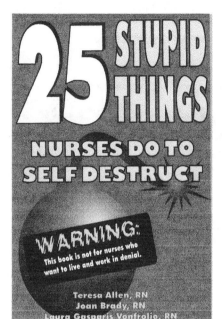

Our hope is that with this book, you will first, become aware of the 25 mistakes that have put nurses into the vulnerable position we are now in. Second, that it will provide guidelines to correct these 25 mistakes. It is only then that we can transform nursing into the rewarding profession it was meant to be.

Allen, Brady and Gasparis-Vonfrolio are armed with experience and should be considered extremely dangerous to the status quo.

They are the public's most ardent advocate, the staff nurse's staunchest ally, and hospital administration's worst nightmare!

Thank you, thank you for putting into words what I've been thinking for 20 years in nursing!

K. Karra Chicago, Il

ONLY
$19⁹⁵
+ $2.50 S/H

Table of Contents

Call 1-800-331-6534
& Charge To MC/VISA

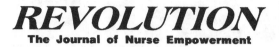
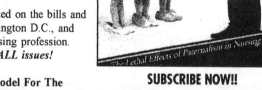

REVOLUTION - The Journal of Nurse Empowerment Presents

The Best of Revolution

OVER 160 PAGES OF GREAT ARTICLES
FROM WINTER 1991-WINTER 1993
OVER 45 GREAT ARTICLES WRITTEN BY
FABULOUS AUTHORS!

SAMPLE ARTICLES

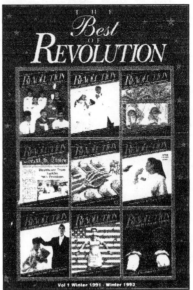

- *"Daddy's Little Girl - The Lethal Effects of Paternilism in Nursing"*
- *"Hospital Practices That Erode Nursing Power"*
- *"How Feminist Philosophy Influences Nursing"*
- *"Codependency: A Nursing Dilemma"*
- *"The Nurse Who Doesn't Exist: Omission and Neglect of Nurses in the Media"*
- *"Why Doesn't A Smart Girl Like You Go To Medical School?"*
- *"POWERQUAKE! The Registered Nurses as Independent Contractor"*
- *"Floating - Do As Your Told"*
- *"Short Staffed and Working Scared - Can Nurses Just Say No?"*

ORDER NOW!
$10.00
for our subscribers

$15.00
for non-subscribers